Contributions to Psychology and Medicine

Contributions to Psychology and Medicine

The Psychology of Childhood Illness
Christine Eiser

Psychological Aspects of Early Breast Cancer
Colette Ray/Michael Baum

Medical Thinking: The Psychology of Medical Judgment and Decision Making
Steven Schwartz/Timothy Griffin

Women With Cancer: Psychological Perspectives
Barbara L. Andersen, Editor

The Somatizing Child: Diagnosis and Treatment of Conversion and Somatization Disorders
Elsa G. Shapiro/Alvin A Rosenfeld

Elsa G. Shapiro
Alvin A Rosenfeld

The Somatizing Child

Diagnosis and Treatment of Conversion and Somatization Disorders

With Contributions by Norman Cohen,
Dorothy A. Levine, and Bruce Renken

Springer-Verlag
New York Berlin Heidelberg
London Paris Tokyo

Dr. Elsa Shapiro
Division of Pediatric Neurology
University of Minnesota
Minneapolis, Minnesota 55455
U.S.A.

Dr. Alvin A Rosenfeld
Senior Research Scholar
Elbenwood Center for the Study
of the Family as Educator
Director, Psychiatric Services
Jewish Child Care Association of New York
New York, New York 10022
U.S.A.

Advisor
J. Richard Eiser
Department of Psychology
University of Exeter
Exeter EX4 4QG
England

Library of Congress Cataloging in Publication Data
Shapiro, Elsa G.
The somatizing child. Diagnosis and treatment of
conversion and somatization disorders.
(Contributions to psychology and medicine)
Bibliography: p.
Includes index.
1. Somatoform disorders in children. I. Rosenfeld,
Alvin A. II. Title. III. Series.
RJ506.S66S53 1986 618.92'8524 86-13037

Softcover reprint of the hardcover 1st edition 1987

Typeset by Publishers Service, Bozeman, Montana

9 8 7 6 5 4 3 2 1

ISBN-13:978-1-4613-8679-7 e-ISBN-13:978-1-4613-8677-3
DOI: 10.1007/978-1-4613-8677-3

In honor of
Minna Shapiro, Jack and Sara Lee Rosenfeld,
and Eli Levine,
and in loving memory of
Solomon Shapiro and Claire Levine

Preface

In the spring of 1982, we began our collaboration while on sabbatical in Jerusalem. Working together at Hadassah Medical Center, we discovered that we had overlapping and complementary interests. The wonderful surroundings combined with a warm friendship nourished the development of this book.

E.G.S.'s interest in neuropsychology, cognitive function, and diagnostic classification and A.A R.'s interest in the development of normal sexual behavior, incest and its consequences for psychopathology, and psychoanalytic thought provided a broad perspective on the field of somatoform disorders. For E.G.S., Lawrence A. Lockman, a faculty member in pediatric neurology at the University of Minnesota who has a great interest in these cases, was particularly helpful. Many of the ideas on case management came from his admonitions to the house staff on rounds regarding proper management of patients and families.

When we began to write the book in the fall of 1984, two students of E.G.S.'s became involved. Norman Cohen, then a post doc, was very interested in pain and biofeedback, having worked extensively in the Pain Clinic at the University of Minnesota Hospitals. He was seeing many of the children in the clinic who required biofeedback and was especially interested in those with headache. He agreed to write the chapter on headache. At the same time, another graduate student, Bruce Renken, became interested in pseudoseizures and very ably assisted us in putting together that chapter. We would also like to thank Dr. Venkat Ramani, who was in the Department of Neurology at that time, for his consultation and advice on that chapter.

Dorothy Levine, wife of A.A R., a practicing pediatrician with extensive experience with somatizing children and a wonderful ability to edit rigorously, has put in an enormous amount of time, energy, and clinical experience to make this a more interesting book.

Lawrence Greenberg and Gloria Leon also deserve our thanks for their suggetions and editing help.

A.A R. would like to thank Mr. Howard Blitman, President, and Mr. David Roth, Executive Vice President, of the Jewish Child Care Association of New York, and Professor Hope Leichter, Director of the Elbenwood Center for providing a creative working environment. He would also like to thank Professor Bruno Bettelheim for being a teacher, friend, and constant source of inspiration.

E.G.S. would like to thank Victor Bloomfield and her children, Jason and Andrew, for their patience, support, and encouragement.

Elsa G. Shapiro
Alvin A Rosenfeld

Contents

1

Introduction

Sally is a 10-year-old girl who was brought to her pediatrician's office because of frequent bouts of abdominal pain and a loss of appetite. These had occurred several times weekly for the last few months. Her symptoms and suffering had become so severe that she began to miss many days of school; as a result, her grades began to drop. Although no vomiting, diarrhea, or weight loss accompanied her abdominal pain and anorexia, she did describe sleeping difficulties even on nights when her stomach did not hurt. When her pediatrician interviewed Sally in greater depth, she found that Sally's grandfather, whom Sally adored, had died of stomach cancer 3 weeks before her abdominal pains began.

Sally is suffering from a somatoform disorder, not from Crohn's disease, ulcerative colitis, or colonic cancer. Had her parents and physician not been attuned to this possibility, Sally might have undergone an extensive, invasive, and very costly medical workup including laboratory, radiologic, and perhaps even surgical explorations to find the cause of her discomfort. Symptoms that originate from psychological processes often mimic organic disease and frequently lead to both medical and psychiatric or psychological referral. The term *somatoform disorder* has recently come into use to describe such symptom complexes. Two major types of somatoform disorders are conversion reactions and somatization disorders.[1]

This century's interest in somatoform symptoms has its roots in the last century's fascination with "hysteria."[2] The vast literature on hysteria is a shaky foundation on which to build a more precise concept of somatoform diagnoses. But it

---

[1]Briefly, as defined by the *Diagnostic and Statistical Manual of the American Psychiatric Association*, 3rd Edition, a conversion reaction is an involuntary loss or alteration in physical functioning, suggesting a physical disorder where the symptoms enable avoidance of a noxious stimulus or obtaining support or are temporally related to a stressor. Criteria for the diagnosis of somatization disorder include reported multiple physical symptoms of long duration that involve several systems of the body, some of which have no organic etiology. These definitions will be expanded in Chapters 3 and 5.

[2]Prior to the third edition of the *Diagnostic and Statistical Manual of the American Psychiatric Association*, somatoform disorders were known as "hysteria." We will use "hysteria" only when referring to studies that used that term. We will address issues of nomenclature in greater detail in later chapters.

is one that needs explanation because current thinking and modern concepts are based largely on the pioneering work of the early psychoanalysts. Their studies, case reports, and armchair speculations have had profound impact on diagnostic criteria, treatment strategies, and etiologic considerations, even among those whose outlook is descriptive or behavioral. Thus, we include a chapter describing these historic antecedents of current thinking about somatoform disorders.

The substantial volume of literature written about somatoform disorders in adult psychopathology reflects the increasingly sophisticated diagnostic criteria for both syndromes. In contrast, the literature on childhood somatoform disorders is quite sparse. In the American pediatric and psychological literature published since 1955, we found only 50 articles (18 of which are single case reports) and 4 book chapters on the subject. The published studies of childhood somatoform disorders tend to use diagnostic criteria that are poorly defined, inconsistent, or drawn from the adult nomenclature. Although adult and child categories may overlap somewhat, the fit is far from perfect. Specific criteria appropriate to children need to be developed and validated.

One unanswered question is how psychogenic pain symptoms fit into the diagnostic criteria for childhood somatoform disorders. In adults, such symptoms are described as psychogenic pain disorder. However, in children, pain, especially headache and stomachache, is the most common somatoform symptom seen by the primary care physician. Also, children's pain symptoms often coexist with other symptoms that are more classically conversion or somatization symptoms.

Many behavioral scientists consider hysteria (especially when used as a synonym for conversion reaction) an outmoded diagnostic category that should be discarded from the psychological and psychiatric lexicon. It is unfashionable today as a field of study, and is rarely even mentioned in modern textbooks of child or adolescent psychopathology. Some scientists view "hysteria" as an extinct form of mental aberration eradicated with the fall of Victorian values. They argue that a modern society unfettered by Victorian concepts of morality and sexuality has no place for hysteria and no need for people to become hysterics in the old sense. Like measles, diphtheria, or polio, an occasional case presents itself, but these behavioral scientists claim that the diagnostic category is nearly eradicated. Others feel that hysteria or somatoform disorders belong in the diagnostic nomenclature, but consider these conditions rare occurrences in modern pediatric practice (Hinman, 1958; Stevens, 1969). Current evidence refutes this belief (Goodyer, 1981; Maloney, 1980; Rae, 1977) and is supported by the studies and clinical material reviewed in this book, where we examine the history, etiology, incidence, nomenclature, diagnosis, treatment, and outcome of childhood somatoform disorders.

Largely because of the widespread belief that somatoform disorders are not important diagnostic entities in childhood, their prevalence in childhood is difficult to estimate. If they are not considered legitimate diagnoses or prevalent enough to be considered in a differential diagnosis, their prevalence, of course, will be underestimated. As a result, physicians who observe somatoform symptoms often mistake their nature and, in cases like Sally's, proceed as if the patient were suffering from a purely physical disorder, even after an exhaustive workup has proven negative (Quill, 1985; Schneider & Rice, 1979). In fact, when taken as a whole, somatoform symptoms are very familiar to primary care physicians and pediatricians in particular. Conditions such as headache, stomachache, other pain disorders, weakness, dizziness, paralysis, and malaise without specific organic cause constitute a considerable proportion of their practice.

The etiology of somatoform disorders is still unknown. As in other psychiatric disorders, both environmental and neurobiological factors are likely to be at work. Among the environmental correlates, sexual abuse seems to be particularly important. Recently, researchers have found that some adolescent girls with "hysterical" seizures (pseudoseizures) and other conversion symptoms have been sexually abused. The importance of early sexual abuse of female children in producing later psychopathology is an issue that has been actively debated (Rosenfeld, Nadelson, Krieger, & Bachman, 1977). Masson's recent thesis (1985), widely publicized in the press, stated that despite evidence to the contrary, Freud abandoned his seduction theory of hysteria, which held that all cases of "hysteria" are caused by childhood molestation.

Since Freud (1896/1962) first wrote about this topic, writers on childhood and adolescent hysteria have frequently referred to sexual concerns, incest, and abuse in somatizing youngsters. However, these reports often do not make it clear whether a molestation actually occurred and, if it did, how it was associated with somatoform symptoms. The recent increase in public concern about the sexual abuse of children, the realization that it is more prevalent than we had thought, and the apparent association with specific somatization symptoms have once again focused attention on sexual abuse as an antecedent and possible etiologic factor (Bernstein, 1969; Goodwin, Simms, & Bergman, 1979; Gross, 1979; LaBarbera & Dozier, 1980).

Although emotional trauma may be important in producing somatoform symptoms, its occurrence does not justify the lack of modern research into the possible neurobiological vulnerability of some individuals (especially females) to such symptoms and the neurologic mechanisms producing these symptoms. The neurobiology of conversion and other somatoform disorders has been largely ignored. In the late nineteenth century, Janet, Charcot, and Breuer believed that the easy hypnotizability and suggestibility of some hysterical patients indicated a biological precondition for the development of hysterical symptoms. Freud deemphasized that issue, since to him, psychologically traumatic experiences seemed sufficient to explain the symptoms.

Since not all individuals subjected to trauma develop somatoform symptoms, understanding the predisposing factors will be important for identifying those people at risk for the disorder and prescribing treatment. Further research in the area of neurobiological factors predisposing to somatoform disorders is needed, and we believe there is reason to focus on children. Etiologic factors may be more easily identified in children than in adults, since children and adolescents have a shorter history, more easily identified motivations, and more easily discerned neurologic vulnerabilities. Despite our increasing sophistication in relating human behavior to its neurochemical and genetic bases, it is disappointing that only one study of somatoform disorders in adolescents or children is available that addresses this question (Regan & LaBarbera, 1984).

Many psychiatric and psychological researchers write as if biology and environment were differing, competing issues. Biological approaches are said to address the structural and physiologic integrity of the nervous system, while psychodynamic factors are considered environmental. A presumption runs through considerable literature that structural and physiologic defects can be considered as if they were independent of environmental ones.

This seems to bother the spirit of biology and current knowledge about the interaction between nature and nurture. Biology is the study of a living organism in interaction with its environment. The accumulating scientific information suggests that human difficulties are reflected in the nervous system's defective functioning. Environmental deprivation can cause irreversible structural abnormalities, and abnormal neural organization has implications for how the organism experiences the environment. As a result, teasing apart the physical and psychological components of various medical conditions is nearly impossible as we discuss in Chapter 3.

We are mindful of the false dichotomy between body and mind, psyche and soma. And we are aware that in discussing factors that give rise to somatizations, those rooted in central nervous system functioning, such as hemispheric differences, and those rooted in emotional factors, such as stress, we dichotomize when synthesis is so sorely needed. But through juxtaposing these different ways of thinking about somatoform disorders, we hope to stimulate an approach to patients that integrates endowment with experience. Since our patients are indivisible, the approach clinicians develop and utilize ought to meet both their physical and emotional needs.

Once the diagnosis of a somatoform disorder is made, how does a practitioner select a treatment approach? What forms of therapy have been tried? Which seem most helpful? Do medications help? What happens to these children later in life? What percentage are "cured?" Do childhood somatoform disorders develop into adult forms? If so, childhood etiology may shed light on adult illness.

Although precise diagnoses ought to lead to more specific treatments, the field has yet to reach that stage. When specific interventions are developed for different syndromes, the pediatric practitioner will finally have tools available to supplant traditional interventions drawn from adult work when these are neither practical nor effective.

In summary, this book considers a number of issues. Current diagnostic categories and treatments are discussed, along with their applicability to children and adolescents. Are childhood and adult somatoform disorders continuous? Do sexual abuse and psychological trauma in general act as etiologic factors for specific symptoms? Can specific neurobiological mechanisms which may play a role in the etiology of somatoform disorders be identified?

Chapter 2 reviews some aspects of the concept of hysteria in an historic context, emphasizing the role that sexual trauma may play in the development of symptoms. The increasingly refined diagnosis of somatoform disorders and the biological and psychological correlates of these syndromes in adults are explored in Chapter 3.

Succeeding chapters are exclusively devoted to the manifestations of somatoform disorders in children and adolescents. Chapter 4 reviews most of the pediatric literature. Chapter 5 presents our concepts of the spectrum of somatoform disorders in children, along with a proposal for changes in the nomenclature. Chapter 6 discusses diagnostic methods and includes some data from psychological test results in a clinical sample of children with somatoform disorders. Chapter 7 outlines treatment methods, emphasizing practical aspects of case management. Chapters 8 and 9 focus on diagnosis and treatment of two of the most common symptom groups, namely, headaches and pseudoseizures, respectively. These chapters pay special attention to biofeedback in the treatment of headache and to identification of subtypes of pseudoseizures.

Several important topics will not be covered in depth. We hope to cover areas that previously have not been well reviewed in the literature. Thus, the substantial literature that exists on abdominal pain in children will not be reviewed in detail. Nor will we deal in depth with psychodynamic psychotherapy for children with somatoform disorders.

Because primary care physicians are the ones who encounter somatoform symptoms most frequently, we address this book primarily to them. We hope to help them make more accurate diagnoses, provide appropriate management and identify children needing referral for more specialized treatment. However, we also direct this book to psychologists and psychiatrists, who may be unfamiliar with the range of symptoms, diagnoses, treatments, and outcomes in somatoform disorders of childhood. Some of the guidelines we discuss may help them be more precise diagnosticians and effective therapists for these children.

Finally, by summarizing the status of this field for clinical researchers, we hope to provide some direction for needed studies. We would like to stimulate hypotheses about etiology that encompass both biological and psychological factors, and encourage others to arrive at more precise definitions, diagnoses, and treatments. If this book can serve to clarify the clinical issues and provide an impetus to future research, we will have achieved our goal.

References

American Psychiatric Association (1980). *Diagnostic and statistical manual of mental disorders* (3rd ed.), Washington DC: Author.

Bernstein, N. (1969). Psychogenic seizures in adolescent girls. *Behavioral Neuropsychiatry, 1*, 31–34.

Freud, S. (1962). The aetiology of hysteria. In J. Strachey (Ed. and Trans.). *The standard edition of the complete psychological works of Sigmund Freud* (Vol. 3, pp. 191–221). London: Hogarth Press. (Original work published 1896.)

Goodwin, J., Simms, M., & Bergman, R. (1979). Hysterical seizures: A sequel to incest. *American Journal of Orthopsychiatry, 49*, 698–703.

Goodyer, I. (1981). Hysterical conversion reactions in childhood. *Journal of Child Psychology and Psychiatry, 22*, 179–186.

Gross, M. (1979). Incestuous rape: A cause for hysterical seizures in four adolescent girls. *American Journal of Orthopsychiatry, 49*, 704–708.

Hinman, A. (1958). Conversion hysteria in childhood. *American Journal of Diseases of Children, 92*, 42–45.

LaBarbera, J.D., & Dozier, E. (1980). Hysterical seizures: The role of sexual exploitation. *Psychosomatics, 21*, 897–903.

Masson, J. (1985). *The assault on truth: Freud's suppression of the seduction theory.* New York: Penguin.

Maloney, M. (1980). Diagnosing hysterical conversion reactions in children. *Journal of Pediatrics, 97*, 1016–1020.

Quill, T.E. (1985). Somatization disorder: One of medicine's blind spots. *Journal of the American Medical Association, 254*, 3075–3079.

Rae, W.A. (1977). Childhood conversion reactions: A review of incidence in pediatric settings. *Journal of Clinical Child Psychology, 6*, 69–72.

Regan, J., & LaBarbera, J.D. (1984). Lateralization of conversion symptoms in children and adolescents. *American Journal of Psychiatry, 141*, 1279–1280.

Rosenfeld, A.A, Nadelson, C.C., Krieger, M.J., & Backman, J. (1977). Incest and the sexual abuse of children. *Journal of the American Academy of Child Psychiatry, 16*, 327–339.

Schneider, S., & Rice, D.R. (1979). Neurological manifestations of childhood hysteria. *Journal of Pediatrics, 94*, 153–156.

Stevens, H. (1969). Conversion hysteria-revisited by the pediatric neurologist. *Clinical Proceedings of the Children's Hospital of Washington, DC, 25*, 27–39.

2

An Historic Overview of the Idea of Hysteria

Philosophers and physicians have pondered the relationship of the mind to the body, psyche to soma, for millenia. At least since the time of the ancient Greeks, they have known that certain emotional symptoms occurred simultaneously with physical illness, raising fundamental issues about the relationship of mind and body.

Hysteria, as somatoform disorders were labeled historically, has been of particular interest to physicians and psychologists because the condition intertwines the manifestations of physical illness with those of mental aberration. However, until the end of the last century, the mental and emotional aberrations were considered to be simply a byproduct of the physical illness. Thus, the ancient Greeks thought that hysteria was purely a somatic illness, its symptoms caused by the woman's uterus wandering throughout the body, causing problems because it was not fixed in place. This theory developed because of several clinical observations; many sufferers from the condition were unmarried girls, the bodily contortions typically a part of the hysterical attack were often blatantly erotic, and hyperesthesia of the genital region was frequently present in female sufferers.

This physical basis for hysteria went unchallenged until the dominant view of academic psychiatry was transformed in the mid-nineteenth century. The new view was that "mental diseases are brain diseases." Academicians believed that the best thing a psychiatrist who wished to help patients could do was to study brain anatomy and pathology. By pursuing that line of investigation, psychiatrists hoped eventually to discover specific treatments for mental diseases and thereby to alleviate untold suffering in future millenia.

A great advance occurred in the nineteenth century when the aniline dye industry developed in Germany. Chemical substances became available that selectively stained portions of the nervous system. These tissue stains became powerful tools in neuroanatomists' hands. These researchers could investigate the brain's microscopic structure and trace the course of its peripheral motor and sensory tracts. Many conditions such a strokes were finally better understood; the brain was divided into what seemed to be functional areas. Disturbingly, however, hysterical symptoms such as certain cases of blindness, paralysis, and paresthesias did not conform to the anatomy being discovered in these painstaking laboratory studies (Rosenfeld, 1978).

For this reason, the neuroses, especially hysteria, presented difficulties to pathoanatomically oriented psychiatrists of that time. Many physicians simply dismissed hysterics as bothersome malingerers. But among those who considered hysteria a real illness, two major theories of causation were debated. Theodor Meynart, Freud's teacher in Vienna in the 1880s, thought it crucial that modern scientific medicine preserve the thesis that all mind diseases are brain diseases. He insisted that some small but as yet undiscovered anatomic anomalies would ultimately be found to demonstrate that hysterical symptoms did conform to anatomy. He postulated microcirculatory defects and transient cerebral ischemias as the cause and, in this way, could explain the lack of pathoanatomic findings at autopsy previously presented by Briquet in his famous book *Traité Clinique et Thérapeutique de l'Hystérie* (1859).

Jean Charcot, the distinguished Parisian neuroanatomist who French writers dubbed the "Napoleon of the neuroses," disagreed. He contended that the neuroanatomic conception to which he had been a vital contributor had reached its limits. New ideas were needed to explain hysteria. Not only had Charcot demonstrated that the paralyses that followed emotional traumata were distinct from those with a clearcut anatomic origin, he had even managed to reproduce nonorganic paralyses by putting the patient under hypnosis. If a paralysis could be created and made to go away through hypnosis, could an anatomic change really be causing it? No, Charcot reasoned. And if hypnotic and hysterical states were caused by vasoconstriction, why was it impossible to reverse them using amyl nitrate, a potent vasodilator?

Yet, although Charcot felt certain that anatomic abnormalities were not at the root, he could not delineate with certainty what did cause hysteria. He asserted that ideas, which may or may not be physicochemical processes, can influence organic processes and play an important role in the formation of hysterical symptoms. Charcot spoke of the "psychogenic nature" of hysterical symptoms and attributed them to the abnormal constitution and physiology of those people who were easily hypnotizable.

When Sigmund Freud,[1] fascinated with the subject of hysteria, came to Paris in the late nineteenth century to study with Charcot, he used Charcot's patients to demonstrate that the failure of hysterical symptoms to reflect the actual anatomic organization of the nervous system (the "ignorance of anatomy") effectively ruled out the possibility of some localized anatomic lesion and required an explanation in terms of a diffuse physiologic abnormality. For example, in hysterical anesthesia of a limb, the loss of sensation typically involved an area defined by common sense, rather than by the actual distribution of sensory nerves.

[1]In writing the historical review of Freud's work, we have drawn heavily from the well known research of Ellenberger (1970) and Sulloway (1979), as well as from a work that deserves to be far more well known than it is, Levin's (1978) *Freud's Early Psychology of the Neuroses*.

Freud was profoundly impressed by Charcot's personality and was influenced by his theory. He abandoned his previous allegiance to Professor Meynert's views as well as his own neuroanatomic bent, and began a study of hysteria, particularly its symptoms, blindness, contractures, convulsions, and disturbances of sensation (Lazare, 1971). Using hypnosis as an investigative tool, Freud hoped that a careful examination of the patient's recollections would lead back to the traumatogenic idea. At first he believed he would ultimately have to invoke physiology as the fundamental etiologic factor, because the nervous "shocks" and traumata his patients had suffered were not so severe as to suggest that neurosis should be the outcome. Some of the sexual traumata he uncovered were incidents no more extreme than a young man putting his hand on his girlfriend's knee or a woman hearing a riddle, the answer to which was obscene. Only when Freud realized that this later "shock" had reactivated the patient's unconscious recollection of a sexual trauma in early childhood did he feel he had discovered an emotional trauma sufficiently powerful to explain the extreme symptoms of his patients with hysteria.

Starting with a physiologic bias (namely, Charcot's theory of hereditary disposition) and using Charcot's notion of the power of ideas, Freud and his senior collaborator Josef Breuer made a psychological hypothesis: Hysterics suffer from reminiscences, repressed memories of long-forgotten traumatic events. Freud found that all hysterics seemed to have suffered a childhood sexual molestation, most often incestuous, that appeared to be etiologic of their condition. But physiology was retained in Freud and Breuer's theory to explain predisposition. In their report, constitution was considered immutable and became the unexplained factor; the hysteric's constitutional predisposition, reflected in easy hypnotizability, was her capacity for conversion. Freud and Breuer did not agree on causality. Freud stressed the sexual nature of the trauma, whereas Breuer emphasized the peculiar mental state the patient had fallen into when the trauma occurred (the hypnoid state).

Freud did not simply deduce from his patients' associations that they had been molested. In many cases, a relative of the patient confirmed the accusation. But he saw a number of other patients who had not been molested whose symptomatology was strikingly similar, if not identical, to those who had been. This led him to abandon his "seduction theory" of hysteria.

Contrary to Masson's (1985) accusation that Freud altered his original theory to win favor in the Viennese medical world, Freud never retracted his original thesis that many of his patients had suffered a molestation in childhood. Freud revised *Three Essays on the Theory of Sexuality* (1905/1964) many times in his life. In the 1924 version of the book, 27 years after his supposed recantation, Freud wrote:

An influence of this kind [seduction] may originate either from adults or from other children. I cannot admit that in my paper on 'The Aetiology of Hysteria' (1896) I exaggerated the frequency or importance of that influence, though I did not then know that persons who remain normal may have had the same experiences in their childhood, and though I consequently overrated the importance of seduction in comparison with the factors of sexual constitution and development. Obviously seduction is not required in order to arouse a child's sexual life; that can also come about spontaneously from internal causes. (pp. 190–191)

That last point Freud makes in the passage just quoted is most difficult for contemporary critics to accept: children who have not been molested can have sexual interests. As Freud discovered, the pleasure-seeking activities of infancy and childhood are both normal and sexual. Bettelheim (personal communication, August 1984) wrote that the notion of childhood innocence should have gone the way of the unicorn. Obviously, it has not. Theories after Freud about the effects of molestation must compare these outcomes with the sexual life of "typical" children, a field in which empiric research is just beginning.

Litin, Giffin, and Johnson (1956) wrote that clinicians unfortunately misinterpreted Freud's experience and assumed he felt that all memories of molestation recalled during psychological treatment were fantasies. "We can see now that in years past patients were lost or were driven into psychoses by our failure to believe them because of our conviction that much of their account must be fantasy" (p. 43).

Shengold (1963) found that his patients who had actually been molested did not try to convince their analyst that their incestuous experiences were real. Rather, these patients tried to convince the analyst that the molestation was a fantasy that had never occurred. Reality had been too painful. Like physically abused children, sexually abused children often assume responsibility for the molestation, saying that the fact it occurred was their own fault. This defensive strategy serves important psychological functions (Wasserman & Rosenfeld, 1985). First, if the child is the bad one, he or she can protect the image of the parent as good, and with that, he or she lives in a world that is good or just. Living in an evil world is intolerable for children. Second, if it is the child's badness that caused the abuse, the child can retain the hope, unrealistic as it may be in these situations, that if he or she behaves better, life will improve. This hope, rather than the grim reality of life, helps the child to continue living.

Prior to Masson, many authors questioned Freud's wisdom in abandoning the seduction theory. Ferenczi's "Confusion of Tongues Between the Adult and the Child" (1933) is a well known and excellent example. Ferenczi felt that traumatic factors play a larger role in causing neurotic symptoms than Freud had appreciated. "Insufficiently deep exploration of the exogenous factor leads to the danger of resorting prematurely to explanations—often too facile explanations—in terms of 'disposition' and 'constitution' (p. 156) Ferenczi realized that problems between the child and the other (nonmolesting) parent made the molestation particularly traumatic:

> Usually the relation to a second adult . . . [e.g., the mother] is not intimate enough for the child to find help there; timid attempts toward this end are refused by her as nonsensical. The misused child changes into a mechanical, obedient automaton or becomes defiant, but is unable to account for the reason of his defiance . . . [p. 163].

Ferenczi's opinion raises critical practical and philosophic questions about the extent to which external experiences give rise to psychopathology. Throughout his career, Freud struggled with the relative importance of real-life experience versus the impact of unresolved fantasies in causing psychopathology. That question remains open. But we wonder whether common exogenous factors might not underlie some conversion cases where no documented incest or sexual abuse occurred. In Freud's time, little was known about family dynamics and sexual lives in "typical" families. New theories about family dynamics allow us to consider aberrations in them as a potential common factor. Marmor (1951) speculated that children with intense oedipal fantasies and associated emotional difficulties seem to come from families that are sexually overstimulating and seductive without overt incest occurring. It is possible that some of Freud's patients who had no documented history of actual incest or sexual abuse may have developed hysterical symptomatology because they came from families in which parents sexually overstimulated them, constantly fueling the children's fantasies and preventing them from resolving their conflicted feelings.

To better understand how sexual behavior that falls short of overt incest can lead to somatoform disorders, we need to understand better the sexual behavior in "typical" families (Rosenfeld, 1977; Rosenfeld et al., 1984). Few data are available to differentiate the typical from the aberrant. If incest is aberrant sexual life in a family, what constitutes typical or normal sexual life in other families? Can a conversion reaction be a child's reaction to an overstimulating environment that stops short of incest (Rosenfeld et al., 1986)? Or has the role of sexual factors and psychologic factors in general been overestimated. Recent articles have hinted at neurobiological and genetic differences between patients with somatoform disorders and controls. Perhaps in the near future new theories about the etiology of somatoform disorders will more successfully integrate the environmental and the neurobiological contributions to symptom formation.

References

Briquet, P. (1959). *Traité clinique et thérapeutique de l'hystérie*. Paris: J.B. Ballière et fils. (Original work published in 1859.)

Ellenberger, H.F. (1970). *The Discovery of the Unconscious*. New York: Basic Books.

Ferenczi, S. (1955). Confusion of tongues between the adult and the child. In M. Balint (Ed.), *Problems and methods in psychoanalysis. The selected papers of Sandor Ferenczi* (Vol. III, pp. 156–167). New York: Basic Books. (Original work published 1933.)

Freud, S. (1964). Three essays on the theory of sexuality. In J. Strachey (Ed. and Trans.). *Standard edition of the complete psychological works of Sigmund Freud* (Vol. 7, pp. 123–303). London: Hogarth Press. (Original work published 1905.)

Freud, S. (1962). The aetiology of hysteria. In J. Strachey (Ed. and Trans.). *Standard edition of the complete psychological works of Sigmund Freud* (Vol. 3). London: Hogarth Press. (Original work published 1896.)

Lazare, A. (1971). The hysterical character in psychoanalytic theory. *Archives of General Psychiatry, 25*, 131–137.

Levin, K. (1978). *Freud's early psychology of the neuroses*. Pittsburgh, PA: University of Pittsburgh Press.

Litin, E.M., Giffin, M., & Johnson, A. (1956). Parental influence in unusual sexual behavior in children. *Psychoanalytic Quarterly, 25*, 37–55.

Marmor, J. (1951). Orality in the hysterical personality. *Journal of the American Psychoanalytic Association, 1*, 656–676.

Masson, J. (1985). *The assault on truth: Freud's suppression of the seduction theory.* New York: Penguin.

Rosenfeld, A.A (1978). Historical perspective on the psychiatric study of incest. *American Journal of Forensic Psychiatry, 1*, 64–79.

Rosenfeld, A.A (1977). Sexual misuse and the family. *Victimology: An International Journal, 2*, 226–235.

Rosenfeld, A.A, Bailey, R., Siegel, B., & Bailey, G. (1986). Delineating incest: Frequency of children touching parents' genitals in a non-clinical population. *Journal of the American Academy of Child Psychiatry, 25*, 481–484.

Rosenfeld, A.A, Siegel-Gorelick, B., Haavik, D., Duryea, M., Wenegrat, A., Martin, J., & Bailey, R. (1984). Parental perceptions of childrens modesty: A cross-sectional survey of ages two to ten years. *Psychiatry, 47*, 351–365.

Shengold, L. (1963). The parent as sphinx. *Journal of the American Psychoanalytic Association, 11*, 725–751.

Sulloway, F. (1979). *Freud: Biologist of the mind.* New York: Basic Books.

Wasserman, S., & Rosenfeld, A.A (1985). Decision-making in child abuse and neglect. *Bulletin of the American Academy of Psychiatry and Law, 13*, 259–271.

3

Somatoform Disorders in Adults: Diagnosis and Predisposition

Many of the diseases plaguing humanity cannot be placed easily in either of the two simple categories of physical and mental illness. In fact, most fall somewhere between the two endpoints of purely physical disease and purely mental or emotional illness. The severity of illness and its expression in any individual are dependent on many factors. These include the person's genetic and physical predisposition, psychological state at the time, as well as environmental factors. Both the physical and the psychological contribute in varying degrees to almost every illness, ranging from the apparently "pure" physical illness of cancer to the apparently "pure" emotional illness of traumatic stress disorder. Between those two endpoints are the psychosomatic illnesses, the behaviorally manageable physical disorders, and the conversion and somatization disorders. The following discussion focuses on the psychological component in disorders along this spectrum.

Clearly, illnesses of a purely physical nature do exist. These include, for example, uncomplicated febrile seizures of childhood, myopia, appendicitis, and infectious diseases such as pertussis and mumps. If any treatment is required for these illnesses, it involves antibiotics, corrective lenses, or even surgery. No one seriously recommends that the clinician approach them psychologically.

But a patient's psychological state can alter the symptom patterns or severity of an indubitably organic illness, although it does not reverse the pathologic organic changes. For instance, several studies and case reports suggest that the frequency of seizures in epilepsy varies with the degree of stress. Changing the stress-inducing situation or modulating the effects of stress through biofeedback and behavior modification (Feldman & Paul, 1976; Mostofsky & Balaschak, 1977; Parrino, 1971) can attenuate the symptoms. Psychological factors have been shown to affect the risk factors of other physical disorders as well. For instance, people with "Type A" behavior patterns may run a higher risk of suffering a myocardial infarction. Although these infarctions have a clear organic basis in the myocardium's inadequate oxygenation, successful intervention strategies to prevent and treat heart attacks for many patients must be aimed both at maintaining sufficient myocardial oxygenation and ameliorating contributing psychological factors such as stress.

Many other illnesses that appear to be purely physical at first glance turn out, on deeper investigation, to have a significant psychological component. Tension or stress can provoke actual physiologic changes in any of a number of organ systems. However, the same degree of stress that evokes no physical symptoms in one individual may provoke severe symptoms in another. This is presumably due to some genetic vulnerability or predisposition, and is often seen to run in families. For example, psychological factors seem to be closely connected to gastric hypersecretion in people with ulcers. This increased secretion appears to be beyond voluntary control. Even an ulcer patient who is aware that increased stress exacerbates his or her symptoms usually has no voluntary control over the physiologic changes. And despite this intimate relationship between organic and psychological processes, the course and prognosis of these diseases are dictated primarily by their pathophysiology. However, although treating the organic component of the illness is critical, psychological treatments can be very important adjuncts. The goal is to help the patient to increase his or her awareness of the emotional factors that exacerbate symptoms, to develop strategies to cope with stress, and to develop more voluntary control over physiologic states. One example of enhanced voluntary control, the use of biofeedback to alter blood flow in the treatment of migraine headaches, is discussed in Chapter 8.

Disorders that at first glance appear to be primary psychological disorders can lead to physical changes of the body that carry significant medical morbidity. Examples of this type of disorder include obesity, anorexia nervosa, bulimia, alcoholism, and drug dependence. The patient is often aware that emotional problems exacerbate the condition's physical symptoms. However, the behavior often persists because it is a manifestation of underlying conflict or abnormal personality development, as well as of physical addiction. Yet, even these disturbances, which are so clearly linked to emotional trauma, appear to have genetic bases for their expression in a given individual, as new studies on alcoholism and obesity show. Regardless of the biochemical cause of obesity or alcoholism, eating less or avoiding alcoholic beverages can essentially abolish the symptoms.

Yet, although most people with behaviorally controllable physical illness recognize that their behavior is directly related to the physical symptoms, they are still unable to modify it. Many clinicians feel that although psychological support is crucial to the treatment, physical assistance is often necessary as well. Frequently, these symptoms must be brought under external control before the underlying psychological pathology can be treated. For instance, addicts must stop using heroin before an underlying depression or other psychopathology can be diagnosed or treated. An alcoholic in the throws of a drinking binge cannot participate in psychotherapy effectively. And obese teenagers must be offered both nutritional guidance and some self-understanding to try to control their problem.

The conversion and somatization disorders are further toward the psychological end of the spectrum. Somatoform disorders are not a single condition. In the pages that follow, the precise definitions, etiologic factors, and diagnoses of these illnesses are discussed. Their severity depends on such variables as the patient's personality type or predisposing factors, an environment that provides the right medium for the expression of the somatic symptoms, and, in some instances, a precipitating stress or conflict. Such symptoms rarely result in permanent organic changes; treatment is primarily psychological. These patients lack not only awareness of the psychological nature of their affliction, but also a general modicum of psychological-mindedness that would allow insight into the reasons for their behavior. Because these patients demonstrate a unique lack of self-awareness, an unconscious need to retain their symptoms, and a lack of observable anxiety, to maintain their involvement physical treatment may be necessary, concurrent with the more relevant psychological treatment.

Adult patients with conversion symptoms are usually unaware that their symptoms help them avoid unpleasant situations. In contrast, most normal people consciously use or have used physical symptoms as an excuse. Although minor "white lies" are normal behavior, the regular and deliberate use of symptoms, or malingering, is usually indicative of deviant social and personality development or serious psychopathology. The most extreme variant of a psychological illness leading to physical disease occurs in Münchhausen's syndrome, in which a patient who wishes to be or enjoys being hospitalized may inflict on himself or herself physical injuries that mimic real disease to get admitted to a hospital and worked up medically. In addition to treatment for the self-inflicted injuries, such disorders require substantial psychiatric treatment, which unfortunately is far from universally successful.

We must clarify the choice of the labels *conversion disorder* and *somatization disorder* and the abandonment of the term *hysteria*. In the past, hysteria was used to denote all types of somatoform symptoms. However, the criteria used for hysteria were vague and inconsistent, and contradictory definitions in current standard dictionaries reflect this historic confusion. The *American Heritage Dictionary* (1982) defines hysteria as "a neurosis characterized by conversion symptoms, a calm mental attitude, and episodes of hallucination, somnambulism, amnesia, and other mental aberrations." In contrast, *Webster's* (1964) defines hysteria as "a psychoneurosis that is marked by emotional excitability, involving disturbances of the psychic, sensory, vasomotor, and visceral functions." The *American Illustrated Medical Dictionary* (1981) describes hysteria as "a psychoneurosis, the symptoms of which are based on conversion and which is characterized by lack of control over acts and emotions, by morbid self-consciousness, by anxiety, by exaggeration of the effect of sensory impressions, and by simulation of various disorders." *Taber's Cyclopedic Medical Dictionary* (1951) defines hysteria as a ". . . psychoneurosis found in a patient of low vitality characterized by psychic weakness and undue susceptibility to autosuggestion." Clearly, one can see a need for a more consistent definition.

As the preceding chapter noted, Freud at first followed Charcot's viewpoint that an emotional trauma precipitated hysteria, a decision that did not endear him to his less than tolerant teacher Meynart. When Freud wrote an obituary for Charcot in 1893, he emphasized what a triumph Charcot's view had been for a humanistic and sensitive approach to these women's suffering. "The first thing

Charcot's work did was to restore . . . dignity to the topic [of hysteria]. Little by little, people gave up the scornful smile with which the patient could at that time feel certain of being met. She was no longer necessarily a malingerer."

Therefore, it is ironic that despite or perhaps as an unforeseen result of Freud's assertion that the motivation behind the symptoms of a patient with hysteria could be understood was that the term continued to be used in the old derogatory sense. "Unconscious" sometimes came to mean a convenient form of unawareness useful in manipulating people. "Hysterical" symptoms have often been looked at as part of a devious defensive strategy for dealing with stress in which the physical symptom is not simply a symbolic resolution of an emotional conflict, but one that is almost consciously manipulative. In the same spirit, among the many negative aspects of the term, hysteria has been used to connote a pattern of behavior (hysterical personality) that included attention-getting, seductive, and overreactive emotional behaviors. Hysteria has also been used as a pejorative term for "distasteful" emotionality, especially in women (e.g., "hysterical female").

In addition, hysteria has come to be synonymous with a syndrome with multiple somatic symptoms known as Briquet's syndrome or somatization disorder, which will be described shortly. Hysteria has also been used to describe a certain psychoneurosis with a specific psychosexual history (Chodoff & Lyons, 1958).

Lack of precise criteria, confusion about the relationship of psychological and physical symptoms, and associated negative connotations have led behavioral scientists to abandon the term hysteria. Chodoff and Lyons (1958) wrote an important paper that formed the basis of our modern nosology. It distinguished between conversion reactions, hysterical personality types (now called histrionic), and somatization disorders. These three different disorders, as outlined in DSM-III, have specific criteria for diagnosis, which we use in this book.

Criteria for Diagnosis and Psychodynamic Factors in Somatoform Disorders

As defined in the third edition of the *Diagnostic and Statistical Manual of Mental Disorders* (DSM III) of the American Psychiatric Association (1980), a conversion disorder (or hysterical neurosis, conversion type) must meet the following criteria:

A. The predominant disturbance is a loss of or alteration in physical functioning suggesting a physical disorder.

B. Psychological factors are judged to be etiologically involved in the symptom as evidenced by one of the following:

(1) there is a temporal relationship between an environmental stimulus that is apparently related to a psychological conflict or need and the initiation or exacerbation of the symptom.

(2) the symptom enables the individual to avoid some activity that is noxious to him or her
(3) the symptom enables the individual to get support from the environment that otherwise might not be forthcoming.

C. It has been determined that the symptom is not under voluntary control.

D. The symptom cannot, after appropriate investigation, be explained by a known physical disorder or pathophysiologic mechanism.

E. The symptom is not limited to pain or to a disturbance in sexual functioning.

F. Not due to somatization disorder or schizophrenia. (p. 247, reprinted with permission.)

Conversion disorder is the only diagnostic category used in DSM-III that specifically invokes a psychodynamic explanation of its symptomatology. Ziegler and Imboden (1962) note that Freud (1956) first used the term conversion in 1894 to denote a process by which the "unbearable idea is rendered innocuous by the quantity of excitation attached to it being transmuted into some bodily form of expression" (p. 63). Breuer and Freud (1925/1955) found that conversion symptoms disappeared and function was restored when memory of the event that precipitated it and the affect associated with that memory were brought to consciousness.

Engel (1983) stated the psychoanalytic view of how conversion symptoms are formed: it is "an intrapsychic process whereby an unacceptable idea or fantasy is expressed and experienced symbolically as . . . a bodily sensation or feeling" (p. 625). He went on to say that such symptoms develop under conditions of deprivation or frustration and are a regressive way of both relating to other people and gratifying an unfulfilled need. In psychoanalytic theory, using repression as a defense mechanism is a precondition for the emergence of conversion symptoms.

The way the symptoms develop is as follows. An individual has a conflict. He or she wishes deeply for something about which he or she simultaneously feels that society or the individual himself or herself strongly disapproves. The psychological mechanism of repression prevents this wish from coming to conscious awareness. Through condensation and displacement, the physical symptoms become a substitute for fantasies that could be morally repugnant, perhaps a perverted sexual activity (hence the famous Freudian maxim, somewhat paraphrased, that conversion is the inverse of perversion). The symptoms may also be the symbolic equivalent of a traumatic memory. These physical symptoms do not take random forms; they develop as a symbolic representation of the wish or fantasy that is frustrated or the trauma that was overwhelming. For example, a paralyzed arm may be a way of saying, "I want to murder X." Thus, the symptom serves the function of preventing the individual from picking up a knife and stabbing the intended victim. Some symptoms are communications, ways to express an idea that cannot be put into words. For example, when a patient who was unable to swallow food was evaluated, the clinician found that his symptom could be viewed as a symbolic way of saying he could not "swallow" what his mother and others in his environment told him to do. The symptom symbolized the patient's impotence, frustration with his dependence, and lack of control of his life, while obfuscating his rage over his situation.

Engel (1983) stated that the conversion symptom is an expression of a wish, an atonement for the guilt of having the wish, a way of removing the conflict (primary gain), and a way to develop a new and perhaps regressive mode of relating through the sick role (secondary gain). Engel cautioned the diagnostician not to label any condition a conversion symptom unless each of the following characteristics are present. There must be an identifiable precipitating stress, clearly demonstrable determinants of symptom choice, and identifiable primary and secondary gain. Primary gain is defined as that aspect of the symptoms which allows the patient to reduce his or her anxiety by avoiding the activity that produces his/her anxiety. Secondary gain is the reinforcing aspect of the symptom and refers to the fact that, because of the symptoms, the patient has more of his or her needs gratified than he or she ordinarily would. For example, an individual who has dependency needs that are ordinarily unmet will get them met if the symptom such as paralysis requires physical assistance and nurturance.

Although histrionic personality disorder will not be discussed at length in this book, some clinicians assert that conversion reactions are more frequent among those who have hysterical or histrionic personality types. The criteria for diagnosis of histrionic personality disorder are listed as follows:

A. Behavior that is overly dramatic, reactive, and intensely expressed, as indicated by at least three of the following:

(1) self-dramatization, e.g., exaggerated expression of emotions
(2) incessant drawing of attention to oneself
(3) craving for activity and excitement
(4) overreaction to minor events
(5) irrational, angry outbursts or tantrums.

B. Characteristic disturbances in interpersonal relationships as indicated by at least two of the following:

(1) perceived by others as shallow and lacking genuineness, even if superficially warm and charming
(2) egocentric, self-indulgent, and inconsiderate of others
(3) vain and demanding
(4) dependent, helpless, constantly seeking reassurance
(5) prone to manipulative suicidal threats, gestures, or attempts. (p. 315, reprinted with permission.)

Whether having a histrionic personality is a prerequisite for developing conversion symptoms has been a matter of controversy. Marmor (1953) and Engel (1983) maintained that such a personality configuration is necessary for conversion symptoms to develop whereas Chodoff and Lyons (1958). Lewis and Berman (1965), and Ziegler, Imboden, and Rodgers (1963) disagreed. The DSM III criteria do not indicate any specific personality type associated with conversion reactions. However, many clinicians describe an increased incidence of both histrionic and dependent personality types among patients with conversion reactions. No studies have been carried out that specifically address this issue.

Somatization disorder is defined in the DSM III by the following criteria:

A. A history of physical symptoms of several years duration, beginning before the age of 30.

B. Complaints of at least 14 symptoms for women and 12 for men, from the 37 symptoms listed [in these categories: sickly, conversion or pseudoneurologic symptoms, gastrointestinal symptoms, female reproductive symptoms, psychosexual symptoms, pain, and cardiopulmonary symptoms]. To count a symptom as present, the individual must report the symptom caused him or her to take medicine (other than aspirin), alter his or her life pattern, or see a physician. The symptoms in the judgment of the clinician are not adequately explained by physical disorder or physical injury, and are not side effects of medication, drugs, or alcohol. The clinician need not be convinced that the symptom was actually present . . . report of the symptom by the individual is sufficient. (p. 243, reprinted with permission.)

Somatization disorder in adults (sometimes known as Briquet's syndrome) was first described by Briquet in 1859 (reprinted in 1959) and elaborated by Guze (1967). According to Guze, it is a syndrome that starts early, occurs mainly in women, and is characterized by multiple recurrent symptoms in many bodily systems. It is a chronic illness without remissions. In this disorder, symptoms are not limited to pseudoneurologic disorders; menstrual disorders, headaches, and stomachaches are frequently seen. Patients with this disorder have often been subjected to an excessive number of surgical procedures.

Somatization disorder may also be associated with histrionic and antisocial personality disorders (Cloninger, Reich, & Guze, 1975; Spalt, 1980). Recent studies (Bohman, Cloninger, von Knorring, & Sigvardsson, 1984; Cloninger, Sigvardsson, von Knorring, & Bohman, 1984; Sigvardsson, von Knorring, Bohman, & Cloninger, 1984) suggest a genetic relationship to both alcoholism and criminality. Daughters of alcoholic criminal fathers, adopted and reared away from their natural parents, had a higher risk for somatoform disorders (compared with nonadopted matched controls). Two distinct types were found among the daughters. A high frequency somatizer was associated with criminal fathers, and a diversiform type of somatizer was associated with alcoholism in the father (Bohman et al., 1984). Although twin studies have found only a modest concordance (Inouye, 1972; Torgersen, 1986), evidence for a high incidence of anxiety disorders in co-twins of individuals with somatoform disorders has been found (Torgersen, 1986).

Although the association of somatization disorder, alcoholism, and antisocial behavior could result from a general chaotic family life-style with many socio-psychological problems including sexual abuse and maltreatment, this does not minimize the importance of the role that genetics may play in transmission of the predisposition to somatoform symptoms. Future research needs to address this issue, especially in children, and to determine more specifically the relative contributions of nature and nuture.

Two other somatoform disorders can be found in the DSM III. Hypochondriasis is described as an "unrealistic interpretation of physical sensations as abnormal, leading to preoccupation with the fear or belief of having a serious disease," not substantiated by physical evaluation, persisting despite reassurance, and impairing functioning. Hypochondriasis is a disorder of middle age, slightly more prevalent in women, and closely tied to depression and anxiety (Barsky, Wyshak, & Klerman, 1986). Since no cases have been described in children as far as we know, it will not be addressed further.

The criteria for psychogenic pain disorder include severe and prolonged pain that is inconsistent in its location with neuroanatomy and an absence of organic findings. In addition, psychological factors are judged causative because of a temporal relationship of an emotional stimulus to the symptom onset or the symptom enables avoidance of an undesirable activity or enhances environmental support. In adults, psychogenic pain disorder can only be distinguished from conversion disorder by the presence of pain instead of other pseudoneurologic symptoms and by its higher incidence. Often, both pain and conversion symptoms coexist in children, and choice of diagnosis is arbitrary. A discussion of a case with this diagnostic dilemma can be found in Spiegel and Shapiro (1985).

Neurobiological Factors in Somatoform Disorders

At what point in the cycle of sensory processing and response does the breakdown occur that leads to conversion symptoms? Is it cortical? If so, can it be localized? Is it at the level of registering sensory input? Is the central regulation of afferent stimuli dysfunctional? How can the experiences that precipitate the illness limit normal awareness of sensory input? What cortical efferent pathways inhibit normal awareness? Answering these and other important neurobiological questions will shed light on how somatoform disorders develop.

But before the neural basis of that predisposition can be delineated, the behavioral abnormalities associated with somatoform disorders must be defined. Is there a defect in attention or selective attention (in particular, attention to endogenous somatic signals)? Is there a defect in affective processing? If so, is it in affective recognition, expression, or experience? Are there cognitive deficits associated with somatoform disorders? Do such patients show indifference to their symptoms?

Many theories incorporate predisposing factors in attempting to explain the mechanism of conversion symptoms. In her comprehensive review of conversion reactions, Jones (1980) pointed out that all theoretical formulations, whether neurophysiologic, behavioral, or psychodynamic, include inhibition of response to sensory input as a major component. The neurophysiologic point of view postulates a cortical inhibition of sensory stimulation at the level of the reticular activating system. Behaviorists see conversion symptoms as reinforced behavior that inhibits, conflicts with, or enables the patient to avoid unpleasant feelings. On the other hand, the psychodynamic point of view states that repression and conversion are manifestations of inhibition by the perceptual apparatus that dampen the anxiety surrounding unacceptable impulses.

Neurophysiologic researchers have used somatosensory average-evoked responses to compare affected and unaffected regions of the body in an attempt to determine if conversion symptoms are associated with reduced sensory responses to electrical stimulation. In some of these studies, a decrement in amplitude of average-evoked responses has been found, which would seem to support the theory that inhibition of perception is involved in persons with conversion anesthesias (Levy & Mushin, 1973; Moldavsky & England, 1975). However, because the somatosensory input and methods of comparison appear to be unreliable and difficult to reproduce at present, the results of these studies are inconclusive.

An excellent study by Horvath, Friedman, and Meares (1980) tested Janet's formulations that the basic defect in conversion is one of selective inattention in which the patient is unable to screen out irrelevant stimuli. Hysterical subjects in remission showed a severe impairment in habituation as measured by galvanic skin response when compared with a control group with anxiety. The authors interpreted this finding as indicating weakness of inhibitory mechanisms.

In reviewing the neuropsychological findings in somatoform disorders, Miller (1984) hypothesized that in conversion, abnormally high corticifugal (efferent) outputs inhibit normal awareness of bodily sensation and, thus, decrease attention, producing both sensory dysfunction and *la belle indifférence*. In contrast, in hypochondriacal patients, the corticifugal inhibitory mechanism is hypofunctioning, and attention to afferent somatic signals is increased. This hypothesis was supported by Bendefeldt, Miller, and Ludwig (1976), who found that tasks requiring vigilance, memory, and concentration were impaired in hysterical subjects. Lader and Sartorius (1968) found that subjects in an active illness state showed no habituation to repeated auditory stimuli. This also supports the hypothesis of weak inhibitory mechanisms. In contrast to findings in other studies, their subjects had markedly high arousal levels, which can be attributed to differences in subject selection or sensitivity of measurement. Lader (1973) feels that such results reflect consistently higher anxiety levels in conversion subjects.

Thus, attentional mechanisms appear to be implicated in the development of somatoform symptoms through their regulation and inhibition of incoming information of a sensory nature. Ludwig (1972), in a theoretical model of the mechanism of conversion, suggests that attentional dysfunction is the core problem because of the inhibition of afferent stimuli.

If a neurophysiologic processing disorder is actually a part of the somatoform disorder pathology, one would expect to find a large number of neurologic problems in patients with somatoform disorders. In fact, neurologic disorders and conversion symptoms have been repeatedly observed to coexist (Mersky & Buhrich, 1975; Mersky & Trimble, 1979). Whitlock (1967) observed that 64% of his sample had some type of cerebral disorder or head injury, as compared with only 5% of his controls. He has postulated that a release of the mechanism of the development of somatoform symptoms occurs with brain stem injury.

A number of researchers have been investigating the role of the two cerebral hemispheres in the genesis of conversion symptoms. Galin, Diamond, and Braff (1977) examined the role of cerebral specialization and found that conversion symptoms are more frequently seen on the left side of the body. Since this side of the body is controlled by the right side of the brain, Galin et al. asserted that this lent support to the idea that the right hemisphere, acting independently of the left, mediates the nonverbal processes that produce the symptoms. Stern (1977) also found that conversion symptoms as well as psychogenic pain symptoms occur more frequently on the left side of the body.

Miller (1984) noted that people with right (but not left) hemisphere damage are more likely to show "neglect" or inattention to the contralateral side of the body. The right hemisphere, he pointed out, plays a "special role in the apperception of the affective qualities of somatic signals coming from the body as a whole" (p. 38). This is because the right hemisphere, in processing stimuli from both sides of the body, has more connections to the reticular formation which mediates attention and arousal than the left hemisphere.

In contrast, in a neuropsychological study of somatization disorders, Flor-Henry, Fromm-Auch, Tapper, and Schopflocher (1981) found that while these patients exhibit dysfunction of the nondominant (right) hemisphere compared with normals, they differ primarily in dominant hemispheric functions. These authors feel that the finding of a nondominant hemisphere disorder in conversion is related to the artifact of "nondominant hemisphere special vulnerability in the female." They feel the underlying disorder is the "imprecise verbal communications, affective incongruity, and conversion symptoms . . . [which] can be understood as reflections of dominant hemispheric dysfunction" (p. 623). They compare the defect in understanding endogenous somatic signals and of sensorimotor intergration with schizophrenia and psychopathy, disorders that they feel are genetically related to conversion disorders since patients with these diagnoses all suffer from a defect in dominant hemisphere function. But Miller (1984) points out that even if Flor-Henry et al. postulate a left hemisphere dysfunction, they still see the somatic symptomatology as right hemisphere-mediated. In a similar vein, Galin (1974) regards right hemisphere cognition (which may result from left hemisphere dysfunction) as congruent with primary process thinking.

Problems in the processing or expression of affect have been frequently described in patients with somatoform disorders. The term "alexithymia" refers to limited emotional awareness and/or ability to describe emotions, as well as an associated impoverishment of fantasy. It is sometimes described as a disconnection of the affective from the verbal. It has been associated primarily with psychophysiologic problems like asthma and hypertension, but it has been found to be even more strongly associated with somatoform symptoms (Lesser, Ford, & Friedman, 1979; Shipko, 1982).

Hoppe (1977) believes that alexithymic patients directly express emotion somatically through right hemisphere channels. He hypothesizes, based in part on the presence of alexithymia in commissurotomized patients (Hoppe & Bogen, 1976), that because of a disconnection between the two hemispheres, there is no verbal expression of affect in alexithymia. Alternatively, right hemisphere lesions have been described as producing an indifference to symptoms and problems in affective comprehension and expression (Denny-Brown, Meyer, & Horenstein, 1952; Gainotti, 1972). Thus, either a disconnection or a right hemisphere defect might explain the affective deficits of patients with somatoform disorders.

In attempting to explain the relationship of alexithymia to conversion, Miller (1984) stated that the defect is not in the transmission of the right hemisphere's knowledge to the left, but in a fundamental inability of the alexithymia patient's left hemisphere to understand and utilize affective information. The result is that affect is expressed through conversion symptoms. For these reasons, some neuropsychologists speculate that a defective relationship between the left and right hemispheres plays a predominant role in somatoform disorders.

However, the term "alexithymia" suffers from a lack of precise or operational definition. It is not clear if the patient suffers from a lack or diminution of experienced emotion or an inability to comprehend emotion or to describe emotion because of a lack of words for inner affective experiences. Imprecise definitions, poor measuring instruments, and a lack of rigor in alexithymia research (Paulson, 1985; Taylor, 1984) have led to inconsistent results and little clarification of the deficits in the processing of affective information in somatoform disorders. The results of a recent study, using a more rigorous content analysis of speech to measure negative affect, did not support the presence of alexithymia in patients with somatization disorder (Oxman, Rosenberg, Schnurr, & Tucker, 1985).

Alexithymia could be explained either as a defense to ward off painful feelings and emotions or a cortico-limbic disconnection syndrome. Whether the alexithymia disconnection hypothesis is valid or is oversimplified with regard to localization and is a modern form of brain mythology will remain an area of question to be decided by empirical research. Another important question is whether evidence of asymmetry of brain function in conversion results from cerebral damage or from differences in cerebral organization and correlated behavioral style. A complex interactional problem between the two hemispheres rather than a specific lateral dysfunction may be better descriptive of the circumstances that lead to conversion symptoms. However, the need to define some neurophysiologic state that predisposes the individual who develops conversion symptoms to the condition persists among scholars and researchers.

The studies discussed here all refer to adult patients; virtually no neuropsychological research has been done on children with somatoform disorders. In the only study published to date, Regan and LaBarbera (1984) found that in contrast to adult patients, children and adolescents with conversion symptoms showed them primarily on the right side of the body. Interestingly, those children with conversion symptoms on the left side also happened to be left-handed. The reinforcing function of incapacitation was hypothesized post hoc as a possible psychological mechanism. The differences between children and adults were hypothesized to relate to the incomplete specialization of the hemispheres in children.

Attempts to define the particular psychological and biological characteristics of those who have conversion symptoms need to be extended down the developmental ladder with hopes that preexisting tendencies to develop such symptoms can be identified in early childhood. Studies such as that of Horvath et al. (1980), who attempted to evaluate modes of information processing and attention, seem particularly applicable to future pediatric research.

Problems in the Diagnosis of Somatoform Symptoms

Diagnosing and understanding conversion and somatization symptoms are difficult partly because the exact connection between the mind and the body remains mysterious. Several problems can arise for the primary care physician who frequently finds such patients in his or her practice (Monson & Smith, 1983). When diagnosis of these conditions is based on excluding physical disease, rather than appreciating that psychogenic factors can play a crucial role in giving rise to physical symptoms, poor management and misdiagnoses result. The physician may find it hard to conceptualize how an interaction of body and mind can produce such a symptom and, consequently, will misdiagnose these cases.

Conversely, overdiagnosis of conversion symptoms can be a serious error. Some physicians commonly label any symptom that is mysterious and for which no specific organic etiology can be found as a conversion symptom. One unfortunate result is that occasionally a diffuse organic problem initially labeled hysterical later turns out to have been an early sign of clearly organic disease such as multiple sclerosis or lupus erythematosis.

One example of this was the case of a woman who began immediately post partum to complain of headaches and showed an increasing disinterest in seeing her new baby. A neurologic evaluation including CT scan was negative. Thirty-six hours after delivery, the patient was found marching around the delivery floor nude. Her obstetricians decided she might be having a conversion reaction as a result of the stress of childbirth and consulted a psychiatrist. Fortunately, the psychiatrist disagreed with this diagnosis and suggested that further medical workup was needed. The patient began having seizures several hours later, and spent several days comatose in an intensive care unit at a large medical institution. Fortunately, she recovered from what was finally felt to be a very rare reaction to the epidural anesthesia she was given for the delivery. Complete medical and psychological recovery was found at follow-up.

A somatoform disorder is not just an aggregation of unexplained physical symptoms. Certain specific psychological criteria need to be met to make the diagnosis. Careful attention to the criteria involved in the diagnoses of conversion, pain, and somatization disorders will eliminate many of the errors that result from the physician's understandable uncertainty or exasperation.

Once the diagnosis of a somatoform disorder is made, physicians often believe that explaining the symptom to the patient ought to lead to its disappearance. It does not. Such symptoms develop because the patient needs them. Most conversion or somatization symptoms serve a psychological function. In some way, the symptom provides the patient with some relief from stress. However, the patient usually is not consciously aware of the symptom's function. If a physician or the patient's family or peers try to explain a symptom whose symbolic meaning may be obvious to them, their explanation may sound like nonsense or even a hostile accusation to the patient. Verbalization of its meaning to the patient does not alter the symptom's function, the conflicts that produced it, or the needs that sustain it. Therefore, since the patient cannot assimilate straightforward information, cognitive approaches often do not alleviate most of these symptoms.

All too frequently, medical personnel speak of somatoform symptoms as if they were unimportant or even disreputable since they are psychologically rather than organically caused. Some physicians may inadvertently demean the symptoms as unimportant compared with "real" medical illnesses. In contrast, mental health personnel often overreact to and overinterpret mild conversion symptoms, as if any somatoform symptom reflected deep pathology that requires intervention; many professionals do not accept that occasionally such symptoms serve the purpose of transient secondary gain, something all individuals need. Often, time alone rather than medical intervention may better serve the individual, but that decision requires clinical judgment and knowledge of these disorders. Both diagnostician and patient benefit if reliable and objective criteria are used to judge the severity and prognosis of the conversion or somatization reaction and to guide the treatment.

References

American Psychiatric Association. (1980). *Diagnostic and statistical manual of mental disorders* (3rd ed.). Washington, DC: American Psychiatric Association.

Barsky, A.J., Wyshak, G., & Klerman, G.L. (1986). Hypochondriasis: An evaluation of the DSM III criteria in medical outpatients. *Archives of General Psychiatry, 43*, 493–500.

Bendefeldt, F., Miller, L., & Ludwig, A. (1976). Cognitive performance in conversion hysteria. *Archives of General Psychiatry, 33*, 1250–1254.

Bohman, M., Cloninger, R., von Knorring, A., & Sigvardsson, S. (1984). An adoption study of somatoform disorders: III. Cross-fostering analysis and genetic relationship to alcoholism and criminality. *Archives of General Psychiatry, 41*, 872–878.

Breuer, J., & Freud, S. (1955). Studies on hysteria. In J. Strachey (Ed. and Trans.). *Standard edition of the complete psychological works of Sigmund Freud* (Vol. 2). London: Hogarth. (Original work published 1925.)

Briquet, P. (1859/1959). *Traité clinique et thérapeutique de l'hystérie*. Paris: J.B. Balliere et fils.

Chodoff, P., & Lyons, H. (1958). Hysteria, the hysterical personality, and "hysterical" conversion. *American Journal of Psychiatry, 114*, 734–740.

Cloninger, C.R., Reich, T., & Guze, S. (1975). The multifactorial model of disease transmission: III. Familial relationship between sociopathy and hysteria (Briquet's syndrome). *British Journal of Psychiatry, 127*, 23–32.

Cloninger, C.R., Sigvardsson, S., von Knorring, A., & Bohman, M. (1984). An adoption study of somatoform disorders: II. Identification of two discrete somatoform disorders. *Archives of General Psychiatry, 41*, 863–871.

Denny-Brown, D., Meyer, J.S., & Horenstein, S. (1952). The significance of perceptual rivalry resulting from parietal lesions. *Brain, 75*, 434–471.

Engel, G.L. (1983). Conversion symptoms. In R.S. Blacklow (Ed.), *McBryde's sign and symptoms: Applied pathologic physiology and clinical interpretation* (6th ed.). Philadelphia: J.B. Lippincott, pp. 623–646.

Feldman, B.G., & Paul, N.G. (1976). Identity of emotional triggers in epilepsy. *Journal of Nervous and Mental Disease, 162*, 345–352.

Flor-Henry, P., Fromm-Auch, D., Tapper, M., & Schopflocher, D. (1981). A neuropsychological study of the stable syndrome of hysteria. *Biological Psychiatry, 16*, 601–626.

Freud, S. (1956). The defence neuro-psychoses. *Collected papers* (Vol. 1). New York: Basic Books.

Gainotti, G. (1972). Emotional behavior and hemispheric side of lesion. *Cortex, 8*, 41–55.

Galin, D., Diamond, R., & Braff, D. (1977). Lateralization of conversion symptoms: More frequent on the left. *American Journal of Psychiatry, 134*, 578–580.

Galin, D. (1974). Implications for psychiatry of left and right cerebral specialization: A neurophysiological context for unconscious processes. *Archives of General Psychiatry, 31*, 572–583.

Guze, S. (1967). The diagnosis of hysteria. *American Journal of Psychiatry, 124*, 491–498.

Hoppe, K.D. (1977). Split brains and psychoanalysis. *Psychoanalytic Quarterly, 46*, 220–244.

Hoppe, K.D., & Bogen, J.E. (1976). Alexithumia in twelve commissurotomized patients. *Psychotherapy and Psychosomatics, 28*, 148–155.

Horvath, T., Friedman, J., & Meares, R. (1980). Attention in hysteria: A study of Janet's hypothesis by means of habituation and arousal measures. *American Journal of Psychiatry, 137*, 217–220.

Inouye, E. (1972). Genetic aspects of neurosis: A review. *International Journal of Mental Health, 1*, 176–189.

Jones, M.M. (1980). Conversion reaction: Anachronism or evolutionary form? A review of the neurologic, behavioral, and psychoanalytic literature. *Psychological Bulletin, 87*, 427–441.

Lader, M. (1973). The psychophysiology of hysterics. *Journal of Psychosomatic Research, 17*, 255–269.

Lader, M., & Sartorius, N. (1968). Anxiety in patients with conversion symptoms. *Journal of Neurology, Neurosurgery and Psychiatry, 31*, 490–495.

Lesser, I.M., Ford, C.V., & Friedman, C.T.H. (1979). Alexithymia in somatizing patients. *General Hospital Psychiatry, 1*, 256–261.

Lewis, W.C., & Berman, M. (1965). Studies of conversion hysteria. *Archives of General Psychiatry, 13*, 275–282.

Levy, R., & Mushin, J. (1973). Somatosensory evoked responses in patients with hysterical anesthesia. *Journal of Psychosomatic Research, 17*, 81–84.

Ludwig, A.M. (1972). Hysteria: A neurobiological theory. *Archives of General Psychiatry, 27*, 771–777.

Marmor, J. (1953). Orality in the hysterical personality. *Journal of the American Psychoanalytic Association, 1*, 1–4.

Mersky, H., & Buhrich, N.H. (1975). Hysteria and organic brain disease. *British Journal of Medical Psychology, 48*, 359–366.

Mersky, H. & Trimble, M. (1979). Personality, sexual adjustment, and brain lesions in patients with conversion symptoms. *American Journal of Psychiatry, 136*, 179–182.

Miller, L. (1984). Neuropsychological concepts of somatoform disorders. *International Journal of Psychiatry and Medicine, 14*, 31–46.

Moldavsky, H., & England, R. (1975). Facilitation of somatosensory average-evoked potentials in hysterical anesthesia and pain. *Archives of General Psychiatry, 32*, 193–197.

Monson, R.A., & Smith, G.R. (1983). Current concepts in psychiatry: Somatization disorder in primary care. *New England Journal of Medicine, 308*, 1464–1465.

Mostofsky, D.I., & Balaschak, B.A. (1977). Psychobiological control of seizures. *Psychological Bulletin, 84*, 723–750.

Oxman, T.E., Rosenberg, S.D., Schnurr, P.P., & Tucker, G.J. (1985). Linguistic dimensions of affect and thought in somatization disorder. *American Journal of Psychiatry, 142*, 1150–1155.

Parrino, J.J. (1971). Reduction of seizures by desensitization. *Journal of Behavior Therapy and Experimental Psychiatry, 2*, 215–218.

Paulson, J.E. (1985). State of the art of alexithumia measurement. *Psychotherapy and Psychosomatics, 44*, 57–64.

Regan, J., & LaBarbera, J.D. (1984). Lateralization of conversion symptoms in children and adolescents. *American Journal of Psychiatry, 141*, 1279–1280.

Shipko, S. (1982). Alexithymia and somatization. *Psychotherapy and Psychosomatics, 37*, 193–201.

Sigvardsson, S., von Knorring, A., Bohman, M., & Cloninger, R. (1984). An adoption study of somatoform disorders: I. The relationship of somatization to psychiatric disability. *Archives of General Psychiatry, 41*, 853–859.

Spalt, L. (1980). Hysteria and antisocial personality. *Journal of Nervous and Mental Disease, 168*, 456–464.

Spiegel, L., & Shapiro, T. (1985). A case of psychogenic pain. In J.M. Weiner (Ed.), Grand rounds in child psychiatry. *Journal of the American Academy of Child Psychiatry, 24*, 781–787.

Stern, D.B. (1977). Handedness and the lateral distribution of conversion reactions. *Journal of Nervous and Mental Disease, 164*, 122–128.

Taylor, G.J. (1984). Alexithymia: Concept, measurement, and implications for treatment. *American Journal of Psychiatry, 141*, 725–732.

Torgersen, S. (1986). Genetics of somatoform disorder. *Archives of General Psychiatry, 43*, 502–505.

Whitlock, F.A. (1967). The aetiology of hysteria. *Acta Psychiatrica. Scandinavica, 43*, 144–162.

Ziegler, F.J., & Imboden, J.B. (1962). Contemporary conversion reactions: II. A conceptual model. *Archives of General Psychiatry, 6*, 279–287.

Ziegler, F.J., Imboden, J.B., & Rodgers, D.A. (1963). Contemporary conversion reactions: III. Diagnostic considerations. *Journal of the American Medical Association, 186*, 91–95.

4

Conversion and Somatization Disorders in Children: Review of the Literature

Substantial data are available about adult somatoform disorders, yet little is known about the natural history and age-related changes of the same conditions in childhood. Research in psychopathology reveals that disorders that present in both children and adults often have different manifestations in childhood because of developmental factors.

The literature on childhood somatoform disorders is meager. We found only 24 research studies, 8 general discussions of somatoform disorders, and 18 case reports (not including the psychoanalytic literature) published since 1955. As in many other psychological disorders of childhood, exact criteria for diagnosis were not developed because it was thought to be impossible and unnecessary. Childhood somatoform disorders are neglected at the present time, just as childhood depression was 15 years ago when the very existence of the syndrome was debated. Yet today, research in childhood depression flourishes, numerous books and articles are published, and new treatments are being employed. This helped a large number of children obtain proper diagnosis and treatment. We anticipate similar benefits for children with somatoform disorders when appropriate diagnostic nomenclature and methods of treatment are developed.

In this chapter, we will ask questions about the current state of knowledge regarding childhood somatoform disorders as a way to review the literature that does exist. These questions center on incidence, diagnostic criteria, etiology, severity, prognosis, psychological characteristics of both patient and family, and, finally, treatment. If no answer can be found in the literature, we will suggest research that is needed to find the answer. This chapter will be of most interest to the researcher and scholar, since our intent is to thoroughly review the literature on childhood somatoform disorders.

Incidence

ARE SOMATOFORM DISORDERS PREVALENT IN CHILDHOOD?

Four studies have tried to identify the incidence of childhood somatoform disorders in the general medical population by reviewing patient records (Table 4.1). Although three (Hinman, 1958; Rae, 1977; Robins & O'Neal, 1953) found

TABLE 4.1. Incidence of Somatoform Disorders in General Medical Settings

Author	Age	Location	Number	Percent	Criteria
Goodyer (1981)	11.3	Park Hospital for Children, Oxford, England	15/3,000	0.50	Monosymptomatic
Rae (1977)	NA	Michigan Children's Hospital, Detroit	NA	0.19	Mixed mono- and polysymptomatic, headaches, stomachaches
Hinman (1958)	9.7	North Carolina Baptist Hospital, Winston-Salem	28/10,935	0.25	Mixed mono- and polysymptomatic
Robins & O'Neal (1953)	10.0	St. Louis Childrens Hospital	41/51,311	0.08	Mixed mono- and polysymptomatic

NA = not available.

very low incidences (0.08 to 0.25%), Goodyer (1981) found an incidence (0.50%) in England twice that of the next highest study. Perhaps the higher incidence he found reflects the careful systematic approach he used. Although his figure may seem miniscule, the incidence of schizophrenia is only 0.85% of the general population. Rather than relying on the clinical judgment of many different primary physicians, Goodyer went through case notes and looked for patients with neurologic symptom constellations for which no organic cause could be found but that coexisted with emotional distress. Goodyer included only monosymptomatic cases, whereas Hinman, Rae, and Robins and O'Neal all included children with both multiple and single symptoms.

The older studies (Hinman, 1958; Robins and O'Neal, 1953) may reflect the physician's less sophisticated psychological approach to patients. Several authors (Rae, 1977; Stevens, 1969) have noted increasing referral rates in recent years.

Can the primary care physician expect to see significant numbers of such children?

Although symptom clusters that meet explicit DMS III criteria are relatively uncommon, somatoform symptoms are quite prevalent. A report by Apley and Naish (1958) suggests that chronic abdominal pain symptoms affect 10 to 13% of school-aged children, and Bille (1961) reported that 11% of children have recurrent headaches. In an 8-year longitudinal study of nonselected school children in Denmark, Oster (1972) found that the prevalence of recurrent abdominal pain was 14.4%, headache 20%, and limb pain 15.5%. In contrast, in a multicenter study, Starfield et al. (1980) found that 5.7 to 10.8% of children had what the authors called "psychosomatic" problems, which included abdominal pain, asthma, headache, constipation, dysmenorrhea, and others. The difference can be accounted for by looking at the means each study used to identify problems. The former study asked children if they had these specific symptoms, whereas in the latter study, the figure is derived from subjects who were not asked specifically about these symptoms.

Thus, combining pain (including headache and abdominal pain), sensory disturbances, and motor symptoms, a significant number of children, perhaps as many as 25% of the general population, may at some time have somatoform symptoms. Although these symptoms alone are not sufficient to warrant a psychiatric diagnosis, they cause the child and family distress, which is why they require the primary care physician's management and constitute a considerable proportion of his or her practice. Some of these children may also require referral for psychological treatment.

How common are somatoform disorders in a psychiatric setting?

One way to examine the incidence of somatoform disorders is to look at the proportion of psychiatric patients who are diagnosed as having a conversion or somatization disorders (Table 4.2). The incidence among psychiatric referrals varies, depending on the type of service, the setting, and the psychological sophistication of the physician making the diagnosis. Services whose referrals come mainly from schools, such as outpatient psychiatry and child guidance clinics, will see few somatoform disorders. School personnel would refer these children to pediatricians because of their complaints. Pediatric neurology, psychiatric liaison, and psychiatric consultation services will see more cases because the referrals are from pediatricians. Because difficult diagnostic problems and children with multiple hospitalizations are referred to tertiary care centers, these facilities see a much higher percentage of these cases. Some primary care physicians are more attentive to psychological factors and are more likely to include somatoform disorders in their differential diagnosis, whereas others continue to treat such patients as if they had organic disease. A medical staff that is familiar with these disorders refers their patients for needed psychiatric care earlier and more frequently.

Seven studies have investigated the incidence of somatoform disorders among psychiatric referrals. One of these, Rae (1977) studied three samples; two in Detroit (Henry Ford Hospital and Michigan Children's Hospital) and one in Oklahoma City (Oklahoma Medical Center). Four studies found incidences in the range of 13 to 24% (Forbis & Jones, 1965; Maloney, 1980; Proctor, 1958; Rae, 1977), three in the range of 8 to 9% (Looff, 1970; Rae, 1977; Robins & O'Neal, 1953), and three in the range of 3 to 5% (Rae, 1977; Rock, 1971; Siegel & Barthel, 1986). Some studies reported incidence with and without abdominal pain and headache patients in their samples (Maloney, 1980; Rae, 1977). If one eliminates the children with those symptoms, the highest incidence becomes 14.5% (Forbis & Jones, 1965).

While Rock (1971) found an incidence of 9.5% in referrals under the age of 6, no other researcher has reported such frequent referrals in that age group. Rae

TABLE 4.2. Incidence of Somatoform Disorders Among Psychiatric Referrals

Author	Age (years)	Location	Setting	Number	Percent	Diagnostic Criteria
Shapiro (author)	13.5	Univ. of Minnesota Hospitals, Minneapolis	Pediatric neurology in- and outpatients	27/500	5.4	Mixed single and multiple symptoms
Siegel & Barthel (1986)	13.4	Milwaukee Children's Hospital	Pediatric inpatients	27/563	4.8	Conversion disorders
Maloney (1980)	12.1	Cincinnati Children's Hospital	Pediatric inpatients	105/630	16.7	With abdominal pain
				62/630	9.1	No abdominal pain
Rae (1977)	NA	Michigan Children's Hospital, Detroit	Pediatric inpatients	NA	24	Mixed with abdominal pain and headaches
					13	Without abdominal pain and headaches
	NA	Henry Ford Hospital, Detroit	Pediatric inpatients	NA	9	Mixed with abdominal pain and headaches
					5	Without abdominal pain and headaches
	NA	Oklahoma Children's Hospital, Oklahoma City	Pediatric inpatients	NA	5	Mixed with abdominal pain and headaches
					3	Without abdominal pain and headaches
Rock (1971)	9.1	Tripler General Hospital, Honolulu	Child psychiatry outpatients	7/196	3.6	Conversion disorder
Looff (1970)	13.3	Univ. of Kentucky Medical Center, Lexington	Pediatric inpatients	8/100	8	Conversion disorder
Forbis & Jones (1965)	about 13	Univ. of Arkansas Medical Center, Little Rock	Child psychiatry outpatients	29/200	14.5	Conversion disorder

TABLE 4.2. *Continued*

Author	Age (years)	Location	Setting	Number	Percent	Diagnostic Criteria
Proctor (1958)	about 12	Univ. of North Carolina Medical Center, Chapel Hill	Child psychiatry inpatients	25/191	13	Mixed
Robins & O'Neal (1953)	10.00	St. Louis Children's Hospital	Pediatric inpatients	41/494	8.3	Mixed

NA = not available.

(1977) mentioned that the incidences at Henry Ford Hospital in Detroit and at the Oklahoma Medical Center may be lower because they serve mainly adolescents, whereas Michigan Children's Hospital, which had a higher incidence, serves primarily younger school-age children.

In our clinic, which is a pediatric neuropsychology clinic serving a pediatric neurology service, 5.4% of referrals are somatoform disorders or 27 of 500 referrals over a 2-year period. These children range in age of 9 years 8 months to 16 years 1 month, with a mean age of 13.5 years.

Are there differences in the incidence of somatoform disorders in males and females?

Table 4.3 summarizes the data on incidence in males and females. As a rule, studies done in child psychiatry or pediatric neurology outpatient clinics find somatoform disorders to be more prevalent among female than among male patients (Gilpin, 1981; Schneider & Rice, 1979; Volkmar, Poll, & Lewis, 1984).

The proportion of males ranges from 13 to 56% of patients reported to have somatoform disorders. Although this range is wide, closer examination reveals that both age and setting have a major effect on the proportion of males referred. Schneider and Rice (1979) and Rock (1971) reported that there is an equal distribution of boys and girls in younger age groups. Boys seem to be more prevalent in samples drawn from pediatric inpatient settings (Goodyer, 1981; Maloney, 1980; Robins & O'Neal, 1953) and in those with black patients in the South (Forbis & Jones, 1965; Proctor, 1958). Proctor (1958), whose study was the only one with more male than female patients, drew his sample entirely from an inpatient child psychiatry unit.

In our pediatric neuropsychology clinic, 18% of patients with a somatoform disorder are male. However, of 12 monosymptomatic cases (primarily conversion) only 1 was male, whereas 4 of the 15 polysymptomatic cases were male. Most of these cases are adolescent and all were white.

TABLE 4.3. Male-Female Percentages in Diagnosis of Somatization and Conversion Disorders

Author	Age (years)	% Male	% Female	Setting	Diagnostic Criteria
Shapiro (author)	13.5	18	82	Pediatric neurology in- and outpatients	Monosymptomatic and polysymptomatic
Siegel & Barthel (1986)	13.4	37	63	Pediatric inpatients	Conversion disorder
Ernst et al. (1984)	NA	44	56	Pediatric outpatients, specialty clinic	Abdominal pain only, somatization disorder
Volkmar et al. (1984)	9.4 12.3	14 33	86 67	Psychiatry outpatients, psychiatry inpatients	Monosymptomatic
Goodyer (1981)	11.3	40	60	Pediatric inpatients	Monosymptomatic
Gilpin (1981)	NA	13	71	Child guidance clinic	Hysterical neurosis Hysterical personality
Maloney (1980)	12.1	47	53	Pediatric inpatients	Includes abdominal pain
Gross (1979)	16	26	74	Epilepsy inpatient unit	Pseudoseizures
Schneider & Rice (1979)	13.0	18	72	Pediatric neurology outpatients	Polysymptomatic
Stevens (1979)	12.2	33	67	Pediatric inpatients	Conversion[a]
Forbis & Jones (1965)	about 13	41	59	Psychiatry outpatients	Conversion[a]
Proctor (1958)	about 12	56	44	Psychiatry inpatients	Mixed
Robins & O'Neal (1953)	10	39	61	Pediatric inpatients	Polysymptomatic

NA = not available.
[a] Unknown if monosymptomatic or polysymptomatic.

Thus, four factors contribute to the different proportion of males and females having somatoform disorders: (a) age—far more adolescent females than males have somatoform disorders, but in younger children, the proportions are more equal; (b) referral source—psychiatric and neurologic outpatient clinics have a higher proportion of females, and pediatric and psychiatric inpatient services have relatively more males; (c) cultural/racial subgroupings—more equal distributions of males and females are found in studies that include black patients; and (d) differing sensitivities of physicians to symptom presentations of such disorders.

Are there cultural or racial differences in incidence?

Cultural differences may contribute to the incidence or identification of conversion reactions. Turgay (1980) reported that the incidence of conversion reactions in Turkey is quite high; although he did not report the exact incidence, it constituted the fourth most prevalent psychiatric diagnosis in children. It is impossible to say whether Goodyer's findings of a higher incidence in a medical population resulted from a differentially higher rate in England.

According to Proctor (1958) and Forbis and Jones (1965), "cultural naïveté" and lack of psychological sophistication related to low socioeconomic status seem to be factors that contribute to the higher prevalence of these disorders in the American South's "Bible Belt" culture. Although Hinman (1958), who did his studies in North Carolina, claimed that North Carolina had a higher incidence, being both rural and Southern, the incidence among pediatric patients at North Carolina Baptist Hospital does not differ substantially from that at Michigan Children's Hospital in Detroit (Rae, 1977). Our own findings in a tertiary care, pediatric neurology setting in the Midwest are that a high proportion (about 60%) of our somatoform disorders comes from rural settings, but this proportion is about the same as in our general patient population.

Only two studies had black patients in their samples. Proctor (1958) found that 33% of children with conversion reaction were black, compared with 10% of patients in other psychiatric categories. However, 27% of the patients in that hospital were black. Forbis and Jones (1965) found that 51% of their conversion patients, but only 10% of psychiatric controls, were black. Whether these different incidences result from referral bias or true differences in prevalence remains unknown. A study of incidence of somatoform disorders with respect to sex and cultural and socioeconomic factors is needed and should particularly be focused on referral patterns and bias in applying diagnostic criteria.

Diagnostic Criteria

What are the most common presenting symptoms in children?

Looff (1970) studied eight children with conversion reactions and eight children with both conversion and psychophysiologic symptoms (presumably polysymptomatic children) and found seizures to be the most common presenting complaint in more than half of the subjects, followed by syncope[1] (found only in the polysymptomatic group). Other symptoms were hyperesthesia,[2] urinary retention, astasia-abasia,[3] hemiparesis,[4] and aphonia,[5] headache, psychogenic vomiting, and hypesthesia.[6]

In 15 cases, Goodyer (1981) found that most common symptoms were loss of function of limbs and disorder of gait accompanied by pain and paresthesias.[7] Turgay (1980) found that half of his 80 conversion reaction patients had hysterical seizures. Muscle contractures, swallowing difficulties, astasia-abasia, aphonia, paralysis, and paresthesias of the extremities followed in frequency. Hinman (1958) found that the most common symptoms in 28 cases were seizures (n = 13), astasia-abasia (n = 5), dysphagia (n = 4),[8] globus hystericus (n = 4),[9] abdominal pain (n = 4), episodic states (n = 3), and paresthesias or hypesthesias (n = 2).

Schneider and Rice (1979) reported on 39 referrals to pediatric neurology because of conversion; 8 had seizures, 6 had paralysis, 4 had syncope (all female), 4 had pain/paresthesias, 4 had dizziness, 2 had visual loss, 2 had tics, 1 had diplopia,[10] and 1 suffered intellectual deterioration.

In our sample of 27 children, pain symptoms were most common, followed by weakness and paralysis and pseudoseizures. Less frequent were sensory and motor symptoms, fatigue and dizziness, and gastrointestinal complaints. Of the 12 monosymptomatic children, 3 had pain, 3 had weakness and paralysis, 2 had psuedoseizures, and the remaining 4 had sensory and motor symptoms. Of the 15 polysymptomatic children, the most common complaint was pain, followed by weakness and paralysis, pseudoseizures, and visual symptoms. Gastrointestinal symptoms, fatigue, and dizziness were found only in this group. However, it must be remembered that the symptom list will reflect referral for questions specific to the setting of pediatric neurology.

Case reports of specific types of conversion symptoms include sixth nerve palsy (Meloff, Meuron, and Buncic, 1980), dysphonia (Giacalone, 1981), dysphagia (Koon, 1983), and several cases of blindness and other visual disturbances (Costenbader & Mousel, 1964; Rada, Krill, Meyer, & Armstrong, 1973; Rada, Meyer, & Kellner, 1978; Rada, Meyer, & Krill, 1969).

To summarize these studies, hysterical seizures or pseudoseizures are by far the most common of the neurologic-type symptoms. Following these are para-

---

[1]Syncope = brief loss of consciousness; fainting.
[2]Hyperesthesia = abnormal sensory sentivity.
[3]Astasia-abasia = inability to walk despite otherwise normal motor function.
[4]Hemiparesis = weakness or paralysis on one side of the body.
[5]Aphonia = inability to talk above a whisper.
[6]Hypesthesia = partial loss of sensation.
[7]Paresthesia = abnormal skin sensation such as tingling, burning, etc.
[8]Dysphagia = inability to swallow.
[9]Globus hystericus = a sensation of a lump in the throat.
[10]Diplopia = double vision.

lyses, pain and paresthesias, astasia-abasia, and a myriad of specific symptoms such as aphonias and blindness.

What factors determine symptom choice?

In childhood conversion reactions, only one study outside the psychoanalytic literature has addressed the question of the symbolic aspects of symptomatology or the specific suitability of the symptom to the psychological conflict. Siegel and Barthel (1986) did not observe a symbolic aspect in the symptoms of the children with conversion disorders who they studied. In our clinical experience, for some children, the symptom can have a special symbolic or functional quality, for example, the child who was blind who did not want to "see" that his mother was a prostitute, or the adolescent with dysphagia who didn't want to "swallow" orders that others gave him. Although the psychoanalytic literature addresses such issues, the validity of the psychoanalytic explanation and of the psychological mechanisms involved has not been sufficiently validated empirically.

Many researchers have noted that children with somatoform symptoms often model them after family members or close friends. Maloney (1980) reported that the somatic symptoms of 12 of the 54 children with grief reaction in his sample mirrored those of a deceased relative. Volkmar et al. (1984) and Siegel and Barthel (1986) found models of illness in family members of children with conversion disorder.

Is "la belle indifférence" present in children?

Patients who seem unconcerned about severely disabling symptoms are said to demonstrate *la belle indifférence.* Looff (1970) stated that this finding reflected difficulty in expressing affect. In contrast, Goodyer (1981) claimed that *la belle indifférence* was present in only a few of his patients; when present, it fluctuated in its presentation. Siegel and Barthel (1986) had similar findings. Since *la belle indifférence* has been found to be present in several other studies (Volkmar et al., 1984; Rock, 1971), further substantiation is needed.

Do somatoform disorders occur more frequently in certain personality types?

Although no studies have looked at personality types associated with somatoform symptoms in children or adolescents, Looff (1970) used psychoanalytic constructs and described oral-dependent conflicts in patients with psychophysiologic symptoms and phallic-oedipal conflicts in patients with conversion reactions. His descriptions coincide with adult criteria for dependent and histrionic personality types, although he did not identify them as such. In contrast, Siegel and Barthel (1986) found no substantiation for the association of conversion and hysterical personality. Research is needed to clarify whether childhood somatoform disorders are found more frequently in dependent and histrionic personality types.

What specific diagnostic criteria should be used for somatoform disorders?

Each investigator has used different diagnostic criteria to study childhood somatoform disorders. Some include only patients with single symptoms; others include patients with multiple symptoms. Some investigators include pain symptoms such as abdominal pain and others do not. Only two groups, Volkmar et al. (1984) and Siegel and Barthel (1986), have used DSM III criteria to diagnose conversion reactions, and only one group, Livingston and Martin-Cannici (1985), has used DSM III criteria to diagnose somatization disorder in children.

Unfortunately, some investigators have included any physical symptom accompanied by psychological factors as an indication of a somatoform disorder. Maloney (1980) used "shifting disabilities in various sensory, visceral, or voluntary motor systems of the body" with unconscious symbolic meaning and no organic pathology as a criterion for conversion reaction. Such a broad classification may include some patients who do not meet any diagnostic criteria. Lumping together various categories and severities of somatoform disorders muddies the waters and makes prediction impossible.

Some researchers diagnose conversion and somatization disorders by exclusion only (Ernst, Routh, & Harper, 1984; Stevens, 1969). Others use specific psychological criteria to make the diagnosis (Goodyer, 1981; Rock, 1971).

In their follow-up study of children with "hysteria," Robins and O'Neal (1953) made suggestions for how *not* to diagnose hysteria. They warned against using stress as a criteria, since children with many disorders are stressed. They suggested avoiding observations lacking specificity, such as "the symptoms do not follow neurologic or physiologic boundaries," or "the symptoms improve by ignoring them," as criteria for diagnosis. Furthermore, they stated that the association of somatic symptoms with nervousness is an insufficient and unreliable combination of signs. Instead they recommended careful differential diagnosis using reliable criteria.

Friedman (1973) gave inclusive criteria for conversion symptoms in adolescents that are relevant to children as well. These criteria are:

(1) the symptom has symbolic meaning,
(2) conversion symptoms are more common in individuals with hysterical personality,
(3) the patient has a characteristic style of reporting symptoms,
(4) there is frequent use of health issues and symptoms in family communication,
(5) the parents are often overprotective,
(6) the patient shows an apparent lack of concern about symptoms,
(7) the symptom reduces anxiety (primary gain),
(8) the symptom helps the adolescent cope with environment (secondary gain),
(9) the symptom occurs at time of stress,
(10) a model for the symptom is present in the child's environment,
(11) there is a frequent medical history of past unexplained symptoms, and

(12) the history and findings of physical examinations are not consistent with anatomic and physiologic concepts.

Research on children with conversion reactions largely supports the presence of most of these characteristics (Siegel & Barthel, 1986). On the other hand, available evidence does not support the symptom's symbolic meaning and the association of conversion reactions with histrionic personality disorder. *La belle indifférence* has some support, but further substantiation is necessary. No one knows just how many of Friedman's criteria are necessary and sufficient for a diagnosis of conversion reaction in children.

Does somatization disorder occur in children?

The only study of children with multiple symptoms that uses specific criteria and studies outcome (Ernst et al., 1984) found that 108 children with functional abdominal pain met the criteria for somatization (Briquet's) disorder. These findings were considered as evidence that a distinct polysymptomatic somatization disorder could begin in childhood and develop with age. Chronicity of the children's condition was related to the number of symptoms. Another study (Carek and Santos, 1984) described 13 children who developed an atypical polysymptomatic somatoform disorder following an infection. This condition was characterized by somatic preoccupation, depressive symptomatology, and lack of awareness of their emotional state. Using DSM III criteria, five prepubertal children were diagnosed as having somatization disorder (Livingston and Martin-Cannici, 1985). Thus, evidence that somatization disorder exists in children has been found, although this condition differs somewhat from the adult disorder.

What research is needed to improve diagnostic criteria in children?

When adult diagnostic categories, in particular DSM III criteria, are applied to children, an open and flexible approach is necessary. A starting point might be assessing the validity of the distinction between monosymptomatic and polysymptomatic disorders. Research should be designed to delineate those criteria that, because of development, might fluctuate in childhood, and to identify specific criteria that are not found in the adult disorder. For example, research on the following aspects of conversion disorder has not been done and is needed:

A. Developmental studies of

(1) *La belle indifférence*, its incidence, factors that contribute to its development, and its relationship to alexithymia (see below and Chapter 3).
(2) Changing nature of precipitating stressors in conversion disorder.
(3) Changing incidence of different presenting symptoms.

B. Studies of the possible symbolic nature of conversion symptoms.

C. A delineation of personality types possibly associated with conversion symptoms.

Far too little work has been done to understand how somatization disorders develop. With the exception of the study by Robins and O'Neal (1953), which may be dated, Ernst et al. (1984) and Routh and Ernst (1984) seem to be the only one that addresses the question of what the precursors to somatization disorder are. Family patterns, initial presentation, and early signs need to be identified and their implications researched if this debilitating disorder is to be prevented.

ARE SOMATOFORM SYMPTOMS THE RESULT OF STRESS OR TRAUMA?

Most criteria that have been proposed for diagnosis of a conversion reaction include primary gain and the avoidance of a noxious or stressful stimulus. The association of psychosocial stressors with somatoform symptoms has been studied extensively.

In a well conceived research study, Volkmar et al. (1984) hypothesized that the psychosocial stressors would precede the emergence of a conversion reaction's symptoms and that the pattern of symptom presentation would be distinct. These researchers found that all but 1 of 30 subjects with conversion disorder had been stressed. However, when they compared them with 30 control subjects with adjustment reaction and found that all but 4 had been stressed, they concluded that no differences in frequency of stressors could be found between the two disorders. However, since the investigators used DSM III criteria, which require that a psychosocial stressor must be present to make the diagnosis of either adjustment reaction or conversion disorder, this was to be expected. Yet the nature of the stressor in the two conditions differed. Twenty-one of the cases of conversion disorder had sexual stressors, as compared with six of those with adjustment reactions. Discriminant analysis differentiated conversion from adjustment reactions by: (a) the presence of neurologic symptoms, (b) the indifference to symptoms, (c) the presence of school problems, and (d) the presence of sexual stressors in the conversion group.

Maloney (1980) used a structured interview to address the issue of precipitating stress and found that 97% of 105 conversion reactions as compared with 92% of psychiatric controls developed after some type of family stress ($p < .05$). Although this finding may be statistically significant, the very close absolute percentages make it functional significance doubtful.

Several studies investigated negative life events as measured by life event scales in children with somatic complaints. Hodges, Kline, Barbero, and Flanery (1984) found that 30 children with recurrent abdominal pain had significantly more stressful life events as measured on the Coddington scale than did healthy children; however, although there were no more stressful life events than in behaviorally disordered children, the type of symptom was related to the type of stress. Children with recurrent abdominal pain were more likely to have stressful life events that centered around illness, hospitalization, and death, while the behaviorally disordered group were more likely to have suffered interpersonal and psychosocial problems such as parental divorce.

Rangaswamy and Kamakshi (1983) found that 88% of a group of adolescents in India who were diagnosed as having hysteria had significant negative life events as measured by the Coddington scale. Greene, Walker, Hickson, and Thompson (1985) found that individuals with chronic somatic complaints had significantly higher mean stress scores (13.2) (as measured by the life stress inventory of Johnson and McCutcheon) than did children receiving physical examinations (3.7) or with chronic medical illness (4.1).

Not all stressors are familial or traumatic. Sudden exacerbation of chronic stress or stress brought on by developmental change, such as puberty (Hryhorczuk, 1981), may precipitate somatoform symptoms. Silver's (1982) case study of an adolescent boy with an undetected learning disability demonstrates how chronic stress, in this case the stress of repeated school failure, can bring on severe conversion symptoms such as pseudoseizures.

Whereas in conversion or monosymptomatic disorders, traumatic antecedents have been found to be present, children with diagnosed somatization disorder were not found to have trauma or stress as a precipitating factor (Ernst et al., 1984; Robins & O'Neal, 1953).

How important is sexual trauma as an antecedent of conversion symptoms?

Studies of hysterical seizures consistently raise the issue of whether patients who have them have been victims of sexual abuse. Bernstein (1969) presented four cases to demonstrate that pseudoseizures are often the result of sexual conflict and pressure.

LaBarbera and Dozier (1981) reviewed studies of incest victims (daughters) and found that hysterical seizures are present in some victims but not all. They also reported four cases in which sexual exploitation preceded the onset of hysterical seizures (LaBarbera & Dozier, 1980). Similarly, Gross (1979) studied four adolescent girls with hysterical seizures and found that they all had been forced into an incestuous relationship with their alcoholic fathers. Goodwin, Simms, and Bergman (1979) studied six cases of adolescents with hysterical seizures and found that all the symptoms were a sequel to incest.

Base rates are a confounding issue in the relationship between sexual trauma and somatoform disorders. Although conversion reactions have a low base rate, evidence is increasing that sexual trauma in girls is prevalent. Emslie and Rosenfeld (1983) found a 40% prevalence among adolescent female psychiatric inpatients. Since sexual trauma may be so prevalent, the number of patients with conversion reactions who have been traumatized in this way may simply reflect the high base rate of sexual trauma. However, future research may, indeed, demonstrate a higher than base rate occurrence of sexual stressors in patients with conversion disorder. A more detailed discussion of this topic can be found in Chapters 3 and 9.

Continuum of Severity

Is there a continuum of severity of conversion or somatization symptoms?

In a theoretical paper, Malmquist (1971) proposed a continuum of severity of conversion cases. Transient "hysterical" symptoms are a normal child's response to external stresses or developmental crises. They can appear and disappear in response to stress. However, some children in this situation somatize as a defense against the stress; if this mechanism is not interrupted as time passes, the pattern becomes entrenched and specific to the conflict. Repression, avoidance, denial, and displacement then lead to *la belle indifférence*. Malmquist stated that a third group of children develop a hysterical neurosis, which includes: (a) internalization of conflicts without a primary reaction to the external environment, and (b) a degree of structuralized conflict between different aspects of the personality such as impulses and the defenses against them, resulting in increasing hospitalizations with undiagnosed complaints.

As yet, we do not know how many children with mild conversion or somatization symptoms do not come to the attention of psychiatric, psychological, or neurologic specialists. Other cases may be handled by primary care physicians. We found no studies of how typical children with no overt psychiatric condition use somatization as a "normal" defense.

Does the presence of symptoms invariably indicate psychopathology?

Hryhorczuk (1981) reported two cases studies of well adjusted adolescents from stable families whose symptomatology resulted from normal adolescent stresses. Both had family members suffering from similar symptoms that had clear organic etiologies. According to Hryhorczuk, in both adolescents, the symptoms resulted from developmental stress characterized by the recrudescence of strong unresolved "oedipal" issues. Neither girl's mother neutralized the overly close relationship between father and daughter. Both adolescents were described as having had healthy ego development, and when they were helped to create distance between father and daughter, with mother as neutralizer, both of their problems resolved.

Like Hryhorczuk, we have seen many adolescent girls whose sexualized relationship with their father, combined with an uninvolved, depressed, or passive mother, has been stressful enough to produce somatoform symptoms without overt sexual abuse. Usually, the relationship between the parents in these families is strained as well.

To understand when intervention is necessary, a study is needed that would compare the incidence of symptoms with the degree of psychopathology. Goodyer (1981) found that 20% of his sample had no psychiatric history; Robins and O'Neal (1953) found that on follow-up, 2 (8%) of their 24 patients were well, suggesting that at least some children with diagnosed symptoms do not ultimately suffer from pervasive psychiatric disorders, although most do. However, the literature does not provide guidelines for the primary care physician that would help determine how serious the symptoms in any individual case are and what intervention is necessary in that situation.

Follow-up

WHAT IS THE LONG-TERM OUTCOME FOR CHILDREN WITH CONVERSION AND SOMATIZATION DISORDERS? WHAT TYPES OF PSYCHIATRIC DIAGNOSES DO THEY HAVE ON FOLLOW-UP?

In a 2-year follow-up of 15 monosymptomatic patients, Goodyer (1981) found that 10 were symptom-free and the rest had a variety of disorders. Schneider and Rice (1979) reported that 20% of their patients with conversion remitted spontaneously during hospitalization, and most remitted within 3 weeks of the initial diagnosis.

Ernst et al. (1984) hypothesized that children with multiple somatic symptoms, in particular abdominal pain, have a high risk for adult somatization disorder (Briquet's syndrome). Can this be documented? Very few data are available. Robins and O'Neal's (1953) follow-up study, the only systematic one, is more than 30-years old.

Robins and O'Neal (1953) contacted 41 children 2 to 17 years after they had been diagnosed as having "hysteria." Of the 23 patients they examined, 4 (17%) were diagnosed as suffering from hysteria on follow-up, 5 (22%) had anxiety neuroses, 3 (13%) had anxiety neurosis plus another diagnosis, 3 (13%) had other diagnoses, 6 (26%) had no diagnosis, and 2 (9%) were well. None were manic depressive or schizophrenic. Because only 4 of 23 patients continued to exhibit "hysteria" or somatization disorder on follow-up, Robins and O'Neal concluded that the disorder is rare and found only in females. They stated that somatization disorders that start in childhood and continue to adulthood, begin with an illness of long duration prior to initial hospitalization that is characterized by multiple symptomatology, including pseudoneurologic symptoms or abdominal pain and vomiting, and somatic symptoms of anxiety.

Thus, the data suggest that although the prognosis for children who present with multiple symptoms is not uniformly good, a significant proportion of conversion reactions are transitory and stress-related.

WHAT IS THE INCIDENCE OF MISDIAGNOSES OF ORGANIC ILLNESS AS A SOMATOFORM DISORDER?

Volkmar et al. (1984) found that of 23 children with conversion disorder located for follow-up, only 2 had organic conditions (seizure disorder and atypical migraine). Virtually none of the children in other studies of somatoform disorders were found to have organic illnesses. In contrast, Rivinus, Jamison, and Graham (1975) reported that of 12 cases of organic neurologic disease that originally presented as psychiatric disorder, 2 were originally diagnosed as hysterical reactions. Thus, although quite infrequent, misdiagnosis does occasionally occur, and the diagnostician needs to be vigilant in identifying an underlying neurologic disorder.

Associated Symptoms

What other forms of psychopathology are associated with conversion or somatization disorder?

Depression and anxiety have both been associated with conversion and somatization disorders. Goodyer (1981) found that 12 of 15 children with conversion symptoms had an additional psychiatric disorder (3 had learning difficulties, 2 had anxiety, 1 had depression, and 6 had behavioral disorders).

Maloney (1980) found that of 105 patients with conversion reactions, 58% had unresolved grief reactions compared with 25% of psychiatric controls (significant at $p < .0001$). These grief reactions were a response to losing a parent or grandparent as a result of death, divorce, or moving.

Carek and Santos (1984) studied 13 children who, after an infection, developed an atypical somatoform disorder characterized mainly by depression. Their depressive symptomatology included dysphoric mood, psychomotor retardation, loss of interest or pleasure, and loss of energy in all subjects. Sleep disturbance was found in eight children, irritability, fatigue, and weakness in six, tearfulness or crying in five, and suicidal thoughts and self-reproach or guilt in four. Interestingly, this group of children could not label their own feelings when asked and seemed unaware of how dysphoric they appeared to others.

Gross (1979) studied four girls with hysterical seizures who had suffered an incestuous rape, and found that all four showed signs of depression. Three of the four had made suicide attempts, and the fourth had suicidal ideation. Rock (1971) and Weller and Weller (1983) also reported depressive symptoms associated with somatoform symptoms in their cases of conversion disorder.

Anxiety symptoms have also been described among children with somatoform symptoms. Robins and O'Neal (1953) found that children with hysterical symptoms also had somatic anxiety symptoms both initially and at follow-up; a substantial number of them were diagnosed as having anxiety neuroses on follow-up. A recent study of adult twins with somatoform disorder found a high incidence of anxiety disorders in their co-twins (Torgersen, 1986).

While depression and anxiety are frequently present in children who somatize, it is not clear whether these symptoms cause or are the result of the somatoform symptoms. Nor is it clear whether the somatoform symptoms are a transitory response to stress and conflict and the beginning of a psychopathologic condition such as depression and anxiety disorders, or the beginning of lifelong maladaptive coping strategies.

School problems are also more common in children with somatoform disorders than among those with other psychiatric disorders. Volkmar et al. (1984) found that significantly more children with conversion disorders had school problems

(27 of 30) than did children with adjustment reactions (10 of 30). Rock (1971) found that most children in his sample had problems with school performance. However, no one has studied the types of learning difficulty or cognitive problems that might characterize such children or whether the problems are secondary to cognitive deficits or to being absent frequently from school.

Regan and LaBarbera (1984) did the only neuropsychologic study of children with somatoform disorders and found that the location on the body of the conversion symptom was related to the subject's handedness. Right-handed children had symptomatology on the right side of the body. This contrasts with adults who have conversion symptoms on the left side of the body, irrespective of handedness (Galin, Diamond, & Braff, 1977; Stern, 1977). Regan and LaBarbera hypothesized that incomplete specialization of the cerebral hemispheres may be the cause of the contradictory findings.

Neuropsychological research is an important direction for future investigations. In our clinic, 75% of children with somatoform disorders have learning, cognitive, or neurologic problems. These deficits warrant careful study to clarify whether this high incidence may be related to the nature of our clinic or to some underlying predisposition that leads to somatoform symptoms developing. Further discussion of the clinical neuropsychological aspects of somatoform disorders can be found in Chapter 6.

Psychological and Psychodynamic Characteristics

Do children with somatoform disorders have specific problems in expressing and communicating about emotion?

Children with somatoform disorders have been generally characterized as having difficulty expressing emotion. However, no empirical studies have tested this hypothesis. Behaviorists have described this difficulty as an inhibition of emotional response, neuropsychologists as a disconnection between the affective state and its verbal description, and psychodynamically oriented clinicians as repression of emotional responses.

Yates and Steward (1976), whose view of somatoform disorders is more behavioral, reported that children with hysteria often come from families with strict religious rules that reinforce the inhibition of emotional expression, especially of negative feelings.

Maloney (1980) took a descriptive approach and found that 88% of his 105 subjects had family communication problems. Despite overt evidence to the contrary, these subjects denied the presence of emotional stressors. Looff (1970) found that patients with both conversion and mixed conversion/psychophysiologic symptoms had difficulty expressing their feelings in words.

In adult patients the term "alexithymia" (Shipko, 1982) has been invented to describe a disconnection between affect and its verbal description, which is thought to be characteristic of patients with somatoform disorders. According to Miller (1984), alexithymia may result from a neurologically based predisposition to a difficulty in labeling affective responses. No studies of alexithymia have been done in children with somatoform disorders.

A more psychodynamic model would suggest that the child represses or denies unacceptable emotions or impulses. Many maladaptive states can result from this. The term "*la belle indifférence*" is used to describe the overt lack of concern or appropriate worry about the symptom, which is said to arise because the feelings are repressed. The symptom is a compromise; the patient's emotional homeostasis is restored by sacrificing some function. Inner conflict is thus contained. The psychoanalytic literature has a wealth of material on the operation of repression and conversion as defense mechanisms.

Parental Characteristics

How prevalent is psychopathology in the family of a child with a conversion or somatization disorder?

Although 85% of Maloney's (1980) sample had a depressed parent, 80% of the psychiatric controls had the same finding. While 44% of the conversion reaction sample of Volkmar et al. (1984) had a history of psychiatric illness in the family, as contrasted to 27% of their adjustment reaction sample, the finding was not statistically significant. Goodyer (1981) found that 73% of his sample with somatoform disorders had immediate family members who had a psychiatric disorder, and clinical anxiety in one of the biological parents occurred in 60% of the subjects. However, the techniques that these researchers used to investigate parental psychopathology (simple history-taking or anecdotal description) were inadequate.

In contrast, Routh and Ernst (1984), using a standardized interview, found that a higher proportion of children with functional abdominal pain had relatives with alcoholism, antisocial or conduct disorder, attention deficit disorder, or somatization disorder than did children with abdominal pain from an organic ailment. Studies of the families of adults with somatization disorder indicate similar familial pathology.

Are there characteristics of parenting styles and personality that are typical of the parents of children with somatoform disorders?

Amazingly little has been written about the parents of children with somatic symptomatology. Reviewing the personality characteristics of parents of patients with somatoform disorders, Rock (1971) found the family to be overprotective and the mothers to be overanxious. Although these families overreacted to stress, they denied the presence of symptoms in their children. These parents had a history of conversion symptoms themselves or were overly concerned about health.

Parents may subtly encourage symptoms. Yates and Steward (1976) described mothers of children with conversion symptoms as overprotective, and fathers as distant or ineffectual. Volkmar et al. (1984) and Siegel and Barthel (1986) found more models of illness and family dysfunction in family members of children with conversion disorders.

Studies of the parents of young children with somatoform disorders describe the mother as overprotective and encouraging dependency, and the father as uninvolved. Yet the opposite appears to be true for adolescent girls, in whom sexualized and close relationships with the father are described, whereas the mother is passive and uninvolved (Bernstein, 1969; Gilpin, 1981; Goodwin, Simms, & Bergman, 1979; Gross, 1979). Not enough work has been done to assess whether this age-related change is valid.

Management and Treatment

What are important management considerations for the primary care physician?

Physicians resist making the diagnosis of conversion and somatization reactions. Of Schneider and Rice's (1979) 39 cases of conversion reactions, most had been treated as if they had physical disease. Nearly all the children with hysterical seizures were receiving anticonvulsant medication. Never did the referring physician suggest that the symptoms might be caused by conversion.

In managing somatoform symptoms, experts suggest that conversion should be entertained early in the diagnostic process (Friedman, 1973; Oberfield, Reuben, & Burkes, 1983; Rock, 1971). Transient symptoms are best managed by the primary care physician (Friedman, 1973; Malmquist, 1971; Rock, 1971). Friedman said that if physicians have the time to listen to adolescent problems, they can often manage them and thereby avoid prolonging the symptoms. Rock (1971) suggested that a pediatrician who intervenes early may avert the need for psychiatric treatment.

Parents often resist communication about the disorder. Yates and Steward (1976) found that families of children with conversion hysteria may ignore treatment recommendations in order to preserve an emotional homeostasis. Oberfield et al. (1983) pointed out that because telling patients that their symptoms are psychological often leads to the disorder worsening, the difference between malingering and conversion disorder needs to be clearly stated. On the other hand, Laybourne and Churchill (1972) stated that the difference between conversion and malingering is a moot point, although they did not address the question of how to interpret diagnostic findings to patients.

What is the best treatment plan for somatoform symptoms? How is symptom removal accomplished?

Friedman (1973) pointed out the need for a definite treatment plan, with short sessions and goals limited to decreasing dependency on secondary gain. Many authors suggest that conversion disorder should be treated using a two-step procedure, with symptom removal first, followed by more traditional psychotherapeutic intervention.

Rock (1971) found that each symptom was associated with a precipitating event and that symptom removal resulted in symptom substitution. However, other investigators have not described this phenomenon. Some have said that symptom substitution occurs if psychotherapy is not forthcoming or if the conflict is not alleviated.

Symptom removal in children with somatic symptoms has been accomplished in a variety of ways, including direct suggestion, hypnosis (Giacalone, 1981), biofeedback, and sodium amytal (Forbis & Jones, 1965; Stevens, 1969). Proctor (1958) suggested that symptom removal always be followed by abreaction, support, and reassurance. He stated that symptom alleviation, although necessary, results in a decline in motivation to carry through with more prolonged treatment. Oberfield et al. (1983), Malmquist (1971), and Friedman (1973) provide detailed descriptions of psychotherapeutic techniques in children with conversion symptoms.

Laybourne and Churchill (1972) are more behavioral in their treatment approach. As in the more dynamic approaches, they recommend that the symptom be removed first. The goal of the initial phase is for the child to reveal his or her secret that produces the symptom, which they feel is in the patient's awareness. Through decreasing secondary gain by having the parents support the child's giving up the sick role, symptoms will be relinquished. After the child's symptoms are removed and the secret that caused the symptom is revealed, then regular insight-oriented therapy is necessary.

What is the outcome of psychotherapy for somatoform disorders?

Although a fair amount has been written about intervention, and there does seem to be some consensus that the two-step treatment procedure is helpful, outcome studies are few. Gross (1979) treated hysterical seizures and found that in 12 cases receiving psychotherapy, 5 receiving psychotropic medication, and 7 receiving hypnotherapy, all were free of spells by 1 to 3 months.

Volkmar et al. (1984) found that therapists reported that 63% of patients with conversion disorders, as compared with 30% of the patients with adjustment reaction, prematurely terminate therapy. However, they had more sessions on average than did the adjustment reaction group.

Proctor (1958) reported that treatment of only 8% of conversion patients actually continued treatment to completion, although 63% of the sample were symptom-free following hospitalization or brief clinic contact.

Schneider and Rice (1979) found that 20% of their cases of conversion hysteria remitted spontaneously. The remainder required psychotherapy. All but one remitted within 3 weeks of hospitalization after treatment was initiated.

Overall, no research definitively supports the approach of symptom removal followed by psychotherapy versus one or the other alone. No comparisons of symptom treatment with spontaneous remission rates have been made. Longitudinal studies of symptom treatment and psychotherapy are required to elucidate these questions.

References

Apley, J., & Naish, N. (1958). Recurrent abdominal pain: A field survey of 1000 school children. *Archives of Diseases of Childhood*, *33*, 165–170.

Bernstein, N. (1969). Psychogenic seizures in adolescent girls *Behavioral Neuropsychiatry*, *1*, 31–34.

Bille, B. (1961). Migraine in school children. *Acta Pediatrica Scandinavica* (Suppl. *236*), 38.

Carek, D.J., & Santos, A.B. (1984). Atypical somatoform disorder following infection in children—a depressive equivalent? *Journal of Clinical Psychiatry*, *45*, 108–111.

Costenbader, F.D., & Mousel, D.K. (1964). Functional amblyopia in early adolescence. *Clinical Proceedings of Childrens Hospital of Washington, D.C.*, *20*, 49–58.

Emslie, G.J., & Rosenfeld, A.A. (1983). Incest reported by children and adolescents hospitalized for severe psychiatric problems. *American Journal of Psychiatry*, *140*, 708–711.

Ernst, A.R., Routh, D.K., & Harper, D. (1984). Abdominal pain in children and symptoms of somatization disorder. *Journal of Pediatric Psychology*, *9*, 77–86.

Forbis, O.L., & Jones, R.H. (1965). Hysteria in childhood. *Southern Medical Journal*, *58*, 1221–1225.

Friedman, S.B. (1973). Conversion symptoms in adolescents. Symposium on adolescent medicine. *Pediatric Clinics of North America*, *20*, 873–882.

Galin, D., Diamond, R., & Braff, D. (1977). Lateralization of conversion symptoms: More frequent on the left. *American Journal of Psychiatry*, *134*, 578–580.

Giacalone, A.V. (1981). Hysterical dysphonia: Hypnotic treatment of a ten year old female. *American Journal of Clinical Hypnosis*, *23*, 289–293.

Gilpin, D.C. (1981). Hysterical disorders observed in a university child guidance clinic. In E.J. Anthony & D.C. Gilpin (Eds.). *Three further clinical faces of childhood*. New York: Spectrum Publications, pp. 59–64.

Goodwin, J., Simms, M., & Bergman, R. (1979). Hysterical seizures: A sequel to incest. *American Journal of Orthopsychiatry*, *49*, 698–703.

Goodyer, I. (1981). Hysterical conversion reactions in childhood. *Journal of Child Psychology and Psychiatry*, *22*, 179–188.

Greene, J.W., Walker, L.S., Hickson, G., & Thompson, J. (1985). Stressful life events and somatic complaints in adolescents. *Pediatrics*, *75*, 19–22.

Gross, M. (1979). Incestuous rape: A cause for hysterical seizures in four adolescent girls. *American Journal of Orthopsychiatry*, *49*, 704–708.

Hinman, A. (1958). Conversion hysteria in childhood. *American Journal of Diseases in Children*, *95*, 42–45.

Hodges, K., Kline, J.J., Barbero, G., & Flanery, R. (1984). Life events occurring in families of children with recurrent abdominal pain. *Journal of Psychosomatic Medicine*, *28*, 185–188.

Hryhorczuk, L.L. (1981). Conversion disorder: A developmental response to stress in adolescence? *Psychosomatics*, *22*, 636–638.

Koon, R.E. (1983). Conversion dysphagia in children. *Psychosomatics*, *24*, 182–184.

LaBarbera, J.D., & Dozier, J.E. (1980). Hysterical seizures: The role of sexual exploitation. *Psychosomatics*, *21*, 897–903.

LaBarbera, J.D., & Dozier, J.E. (1981). Psychologic responses of incestuous daughters: Emerging patterns. *Southern Medical Journal*, *74*, 1478–1480.

Laybourne, T.C., & Churchill, S.W. (1972). Symptom discouragement in treating hysterical reactions in childhood. *International Journal of Psychotherapy*, *1*, 111–123.

Livingston, R., & Martin-Cannici, C. (1985). Multiple somatic complaints and possible somatization disorder in prepubertal children. *Journal of the American Academy of Child Psychiatry*, *24*, 603–607.

Looff, D.H. (1970). Psychophysiologic and conversion reactions in children. *Journal of the American Academy of Child Psychiatry*, *9*, 318–331.

Malmquist, C. (1971). Hysteria in childhood. *Postgraduate Medicine*, *50*, 112–117.

Maloney, M. (1980). Diagnosing hysterical conversion reactions in children. *Journal of Pediatrics*, *97*, 1016–1020.

Meloff, K.L., Meuron, G., & Buncic, J.R. (1980). Conversion sixth nerve palsy in a child. *Psychosomatics*, *21*, 769–770.

Miller, L. (1984). Neuropsychological concepts of somatoform disorders. *International Journal of Psychiatry and Medicine*, *14*, 31–46.

Oberfield, R.A., Reuben, R., & Burkes, J. (1983). Interdisciplinary approach to conversion disorders in adolescent girls. *Psychosomatics*, *24*, 983–989.

Oster, J. (1972). Recurrent abdominal pain, headache, and limb pains in children and adolescents. *Pediatrics*, *50*, 429–436.

Proctor, J.T. (1958). Hysteria in childhood. *American Journal of Orthopsychiatry*, *28*, 394–407.

Rada, R.T., Krill, A.E., Meyer, G.G., & Armstrong, D. (1973). Visual conversion reaction in children. II. Follow-up. *Psychosomatics*, *14*, 271–276.

Rada, R.T., Meyer, G.G., & Kellner, R. (1978). Visual conversion reaction in children and adults. *Journal of Nervous and Mental Disease*, *168*, 580–587.

Rada, R.T., Meyer, G.G., & Krill, A.E. (1969). Visual conversion reaction in children. I. Diagnosis. *Psychosomatics*, *10*, 23–28.

Rae, W.A. (1977). Childhood conversion reactions: A review of incidence in pediatric settings. *Journal of Clinical Child Psychology*, *6*, 69–72.

Rangaswami, K., & Kamakshi, G. (1983). Life events in hysterial adolescents. *Child Psychiatry Quarterly*, *16*, 26–33.

Regan, J., & LaBarbera, J.D. (1984). Lateralization of conversion symptoms in children and adolescents. *American Journal of Psychiatry*, *141*, 1279–1280.

Rivinus, T.M., Jamison, D.L., & Graham, P.J. (1975). Childhood organic-neurological diseases presenting as a psychiatric disorder. *Archives of Diseases in Children*, *50*, 115–119.

Robins, E., & O'Neal, P. (1953). Clinical features of hysteria in children—with a note on prognosis: A two to seventeen year follow-up study of 41 patients. *Nervous Child*, *10*, 246–271.

Rock, N. (1971). Conversion reactions in childhood: A clinical study on childhood neuroses. *Journal of the American Academy of Child Psychiatry*, *10*, 65–93.

Routh, D.K., & Ernst, A.R. (1984). Somatization disorder in relatives of children and adolescents with functional abdominal pain. *Journal of Pediatric Psychology*, *9*, 427–437.

Schneider, S., & Rice, D.R. (1979). Neurologic manifestations of childhood hysteria. *Pediatrics, 94*, 153–156.

Shipko, S. (1982). Alexithymia and somatization. *Psychotherapy and Psychosomatics, 37*, 193–201.

Siegel, M., & Barthel, R.P. (1986). Conversion disorders on a child psychiatry consultation service. *Psychosomatics, 27*, 201–204.

Silver, L.B. (1982). Conversion disorder with pseudoseizures in adolescence: A stress reaction to unrecognized and untreated learning disabilities. *Journal of the American Academy of Child Psychiatry, 21*, 508–512.

Starfield, B., Gross, E., Wood, M., Pantell, R., Allen, C., Gordon, I.B., Moffatt, P., Drachman, R., & Katz, H. (1980). Psychosocial and psychosomatic diagnoses in primary care of children. *Pediatrics, 66*, 159–167.

Stern, D.B. (1977). Handedness and the lateral distribution of conversion reactions. *Journal of Nervous and Mental Disease, 164*, 122–128.

Stevens, H. (1969). Conversion hysteria—revisited by the pediatric neurologist. *Clinical Proceedings of the Childrens Hospital of Washington, DC, 25*, 27–39.

Torgerson, S. (1986). Genetics of somatoform disorder. *Archives of General Psychiatry, 43*, 502–505.

Turgay, A. (1980). Conversion reactions in children. *Psychiatric Journal of the University of Ottawa, 5*, 287–294.

Volkmar, F.R., Poll, J., & Lewis, M. (1984). Conversion reactions in childhood and adolescence. *Journal of the American Academy of Child Psychiatry, 23*, 424–430.

Weller, E.B., & Weller, R.A. (1983). Case report of conversion symptom associated with major depressive disorder in a child. *American Journal of Psychiatry, 140*, 1079–1080.

Yates, A., & Steward, M. (1976). Conversion hysteria in childhood. *Clinical Pediatrics, 15*, 379–382.

5

A Spectrum of Conversion and Somatization Disorders in Children

We have seen many children with somatoform disorders in pediatric neurology and neuropsychology inpatient and outpatient services (E.G.S. and N.C.), in a child psychiatry setting (A.R.), and in a general pediatric practice (D.A.L.). Before an attempt at classification is made, however, some characteristics of childhood conversion and somatization disorders should be discussed, because such reactions in childhood differ in important ways from adult disorders. Rather than extrapolating from the adult literature or from DSM III on to children, we present categories with case examples that reflect the symptom patterns we have observed.

Etiologic Factors

Organic Predisposition

Almost every child with a somatoform disorder seen in our pediatric neurology clinic has a history of a neurologic disorder or signs on neuropsychological testing of a cognitive deficit, probably secondary to covert neurologic problems. Obviously, this clinical setting generates a biased sample. However, some evidence suggests that somatoform disorders might be linked to cognitive and neurologic dysfunction (Whitlock, 1967). Volkmar, Poll, and Lewis (1984) found that their group of subjects with conversion disorders suffered from a greater number of learning and school problems than did a comparison group of children with adjustment reactions. Thus, the relationship of somatoform disorders to an underlying diathesis may be easier to detect in children than in adults because fewer years of experience camouflage them.

Stressful Events as Precipitants

A conflict or a noxious stimulus within the child's environment, such as a loss, a divorce, or a change in the family constellation, often precipitates the illness. The conversion symptom resolves or mitigates the child's pain and anxiety, albeit at the high price of compromised functions. This decrease in stress is called primary gain. Although both adults and children develop symptoms in this fashion, relatively minor stresses can evoke simple conversion symptoms in children, which resolve quickly if the stress is relieved or at least does not increase in severity. In addition, normal developmental changes alone, such as puberty, may be stressful enough to bring on significant somatoform symptoms, which resolve with time. Sexual concerns have been described as more central in children with somatoform symptoms than in children with other psychiatric diagnoses (Volkmar et al., 1984).

Physical Illness as a Precipitant

In many cases, some actual physical illness may precede or even coexist with the first presentation of a somatoform symptom. Symptoms of a flulike or a neurologic illness, during which the child had previously unmet needs gratified, frequently do not disappear as the organic component of the illness resolves. In one of the rare cases of acute rheumatic fever we have seen within the last 5 years, this 9-year-old female's mild arthralgias persisted far longer than would be expected during the normal course of the illness. As a result, she was able to avoid activities that she found unpleasant, including gym and household chores. In other cases, the symptoms of a previous illness recur with stress. Carek and Santos (1984) described such a somatoform syndrome following infectious disorders. Commonly, specific symptoms of a chronic illness such as epilepsy and migraine headache may coexist with conversion symptoms that mimic the organic illness.

Characteristics of Children and Their Families

Family Communication Problems

Looff (1970) described families of children with conversion symptoms as having a limited ability to express emotion verbally. We have found that children with serious somatoform disorders come from families who use physical symptoms, not only as a way to have their needs met, but also as a more general means of communicating about emotions. Somatic symptoms become the only legitimate way to express emotions and needs and the only means to their gratification. Many parents of children with somatoform illnesses respond to the symptoms with solicitious behavior, thereby reinforcing the child's physical symptomatology and continued incapacitation.

In addition, the physical symptom may be a bodily way of expressing a thought or feeling. A child may have chest pains because his 'heart is breaking' or have belly pains because he feels like someone "kicked him in the stomach." The symbolic expression of an affect is often more obvious and easier to interpret in children, perhaps because they are cognitively less sophisticated.

Because the diagnostic process in children is more likely to involve other family members, affective communication problems are more apparent than in adults. Such data are not routinely obtained as part of an adult's evaluation. Thus, although the impact of communication difficulties is more obvious in children, the question of whether child and adult cases differ in regards to affective expression remains unanswered.

School Absence

Almost all children with somatoform disorders are absent from school for extended periods. Parents who are concerned that physical illness is causing their child's disorder often encourage the child to stay home. The longer that children with somatoform symptoms stay home, the further behind they fall and the more difficult the return to school becomes. Thus, school refusal frequently becomes a secondary accompaniment to the somatoform symptom.

Often, it is the school teacher or nurse who helps identify these cases. The child is not always brought to the doctor each time he or she is kept home from school. So the pediatrician may not be aware of the extent of the incapacitation unless concerned school personnel call him or her to inquire about the child's state of health.

Adult Models

Many children with serious somatoform symptoms have an adult in their family who uses physical symptoms for secondary gain and to satisfy certain needs. When susceptible children see that friends or other important individuals in their lives get their dependency needs met through physical symptomatology, they learn this coping strategy. Modeling behavior in this way influences children more than it does adults with somatoform disorders. Children are more suggestible, more susceptible to the influences of their environment, and more ready to identify with the adults who surround them. Some children develop somatoform symptoms closely related to the illness that they see in their relatives. For example, children who complain of headaches often have family members with frequent incapacitating headaches.

Symptom Awareness

Children are often more aware than adults are of their symptom's psychological function. This awareness can coexist with the presence of the symptom without indicating malingering. Formerly, some believed that when the conflict was brought to the child's conscious awareness, the symptom would disappear as it usually does in adults. In contrast, Laybourne and Churchill (1972) state that the child is always aware of the symptom's meaning, but because it is unverbalized, it produces the symptom. They feel verbalization is sufficient for symptom cure. However, in many cases, we have observed that awareness is not sufficient to cure the symptom. The conflict and stress producing the symptom and the secondary gain from the symptom, not its lack of consciousness, seem to perpetuate it. Perhaps conscious and unconscious processes are less well demarcated in children. The heightened suggestibility, easier hypnotizability, and readier access to fantasy through play in preadolescent children as compared with adults support this hypothesis.

Associated Symptoms

Children with somatoform disorders are frequently depressed and anxious. Depression and anxiety may be the result or the cause of the somatoform symptom. This is especially likely in cases where the child's symptom has become the focus of family communication or where multiple symptoms are persistent. In contrast, we have observed that in mild polysymptomatic cases and in some conversion cases, premorbid adjustments are often described as good, and they continue to be so after the symptoms have resolved.

Symptom Instability

Because children somatize frequently, conversion symptoms do not necessarily imply a dire prognosis. Conversion symptoms can arise from specific developmental stresses and disappear spontaneously shortly after they appear. Follow-up studies indicate a high incidence of spontaneous remission (Goodyer, 1981; Schneider & Rice, 1979). The symptoms are fluid and, in many cases, easily influenced by environmental factors because children are suggestible and the child's psychopathology is not entrenched the way it might be in an adult. This fluidity sometimes leads parents or physicians to mistake conversion symptoms for the conscious act of malingering.

Demographic Factors

Cultural and Social Background

Somatoform symptoms have been said to be more common in children from low socioeconomic, rural and poor educational backgrounds (Forbis & Jones, 1965; Hinman, 1958; Proctor, 1958). An overabundance of the somatizing children seen in our pediatric neurology cases come from rural or low socioeconomic settings in Minnesota where psychological-mindedness is relatively absent. Parents from poor socioeconomic backgrounds may find the fact that their child suffers from an organic disease easier to understand than that the symptoms are caused by emotional distress or conflict. Hinman (1958) has called this "cultural naiveté." However, we have observed that younger children with somatoform symptoms come from a wider range of socioeconomic and cultural backgrounds.

Sex Ratios

Among prepubertal children, boys and girls suffer these symptoms with almost equal frequency (Goodyer, 1981; Maloney, 1980). After puberty, the frequency increases among girls and decreases or remains the same among boys. Among adults, conversion reactions and somatization disorders that come to professional attention are far more common in women (Woodruff, Clayton, & Guze, 1969). Women may actually suffer these ailments more frequently, perhaps as a result of sexual abuse, but other explanations may also account for the disparity. Perhaps this disparity results from our culture's traditional tendency to teach women to internalize their feelings, whereas men are more often encouraged to express feelings, especially aggressive or sexual ones, more externally. It may also be the result of our culture's attitude that men should not focus on or complain about physical symptoms. Diagnostic bias may also be an important factor in sex ratios. Even when no organic cause can be found for a postpubescent young man's physical symptom and the necessary psychological criteria are met, some physicians are reluctant to diagnose the condition as a conversion symptom, perhaps still believing the old-fashioned psychological myths that hysteria occurs only in females.

The Spectrum of Somatoform Disorders

Somatoform symptoms in children fall along a clinical spectrum, some of whose nodal points will be described with clinical examples. The spectrum is not necessarily continuous, but the lack of attention in DSM III to the broad range of somatoform disorders in children and the differing presentations of conversion reactions and somatization disorders in childhood led us to develop this categorization. They range from transitory reactions of childhood to early manifestations of disorders that become defined only during adulthood.

The relationship among these various types and their relative severity is unclear. Although retrospective histories of individual cases sometimes suggest that more severe situations started out as less serious ones, we know of no evidence indicating that, if not attended to, mild conditions routinely progress to severe ones. In fact, many somatoform symptoms in children resolve spontaneously. However, the pediatrician's and primary care physician's thoughtful interventions can help prevent symptoms from becoming more entrenched or taking longer to resolve.

Nonspecific Transient Stress Avoiders (Normal Type)

A psychiatric diagnosis should not be assigned to symptoms of this type. Nonspecific symptoms like headache, stomachache, and malaise occur in all children as ways to avoid specific stress. For instance, many children get a headache at one time or another to avoid going to school. In normal children in adequate environments, these symptoms are recognized for what they are and if handled in a matter of fact way, they resolve quickly. Sensitivity to the child's concerns and needs combined with limit setting is usually helpful. For instance, the child's concerns regarding school should be discussed, and he or she should be reassured and then sent to school. Unless the family focuses on these somatic symptoms, they do not usually progress. As the stress the child is avoiding diminishes or disappears, the symptoms resolve. Many children with unfavorable school environments, teachers they do not get along with, or work they are unable to do may develop somatic symptoms as an indirect means of resisting to go to school. If parents insist that the child attend school, the symptoms often resolve by midmorning.

John is a 7½-year-old second grade boy with a previously diagnosed mild learning disability of an auditory-processing type. After the winter holiday from school, John began to complain about stomachaches upon waking in the morning. Concerned that John might be ill, his mother allowed him to stay home that morning. She noticed that he was fine after an hour or two, and so she sent him to school at midday. He had no symptoms. The next morning he again complained about a stomachache, but his mother sent him to school anyway. When he arrived at school, he complained about his stomachache and was allowed to stay in the nurse's office for a short period of time, after which he returned to class. The nurse, being astute, checked and found that the class he was missing was reading. She called John's mother, who asked John whether something about this class was bothering him. John replied that a few weeks earlier the children had started to read aloud in class. Since he was struggling in the lowest reading group in his regular class, he was embarrassed to read aloud in front of others who read so much better. When the mother pointed this out, John's teacher agreed not to ask him to read aloud. She was also encouraged to check with his special learning disability teacher when changing her expectations of his work. John's symptoms did not recur.

In this case, the symptom is primarily a stress avoider. The symptom did not persist after the stress was eliminated. The nurse was sensitive to John's needs, as were his mother and teacher, who were already giving him special help for his reading disability. John's mother handled the situation appropriately and focused not on the symptom, but on its cause. The environmental stress was noted and resolved, and no secondary gain reinforced the symptoms.

Mild Polysymptomatic Somatization Disorder (Type 1)

Children with this disorder miss school or activities frequently because of a number of different symptoms such as headache or stomachache. In these cases, symptoms are rather vague and nonspecific, with malaise and various types of pain being the most common complaints. They are signs neither of serious childhood psychopathology nor of conscious manipulation. These children have symptoms that persist and recur because in those families, illness is a permissible way to express emotions, a way to ask for and receive indulgence and affection. Because the parents do not recognize the symptom for what it is, they can neither help alleviate the stress that underlies the symptom, nor set firm limits on time missed because of the symptom. They may focus on somatic symptoms because they themselves have had their needs met by being ill.

Without intervention, many of these cases persist and intensify. Psychopathology develops insidiously.

Kathy is an attractive 14-year-old adolescent who was hospitalized on the pediatric neurology service because of severe, unremitting headache, including persistent pain in the center of her head of a month's duration. As a small child, she had had Reye's syndrome, and since that time she has had occasional migraine but no other neurologic sequelae. The pain began when she became very stressed while preparing for a party to which she had invited her friends, some of whom, to her dismay, were unable to attend. Since then, she has had the pain even at night. It woke her and prevented her from attending school, which provided her with home-bound instruction. This was her second hospitalization, having been worked up at another medical center where her symptoms were identified as stress-related, and biofeedback was recommended. She tried this treatment and found that it helped her only minimally.

All neurologic examinations including CT scan, magnetic resonance imaging, and EEG were negative. Kathy was well groomed, dressed in a fashion considered mature for her age, spoke articulately, and expressed distress only when she was asked specifically about her headaches. An interview revealed that prior to this illness, Kathy had been a socially well-adjusted adolescent with some fears about having a brain tumor or some other sequelae to her Reye's syndrome. Other than that fear, she demonstrated little overt distress.

Since her episode of Reye's syndrome, Kathy's parents had perceived her as fragile. They reported that she has always been a dependent child and was always getting sick. When Kathy was 10, she was hospitalized for stomachaches. All tests at that time were negative. Two years later, a laparoscopy was performed after complaining about menstrual pain. An adhesion was diagnosed.

Kathy's father is gregarious, focuses on Kathy's somatic functions to an unusual extent, and dotes on her, encouraging her dependency. Her mother is somewhat withdrawn and does not interfere with the very close father-daughter relationship, although she does report being close to Kathy and seems to be reinforcing Kathy's somatic symptoms. By description, Kathy's grandmother has either Briquet's syndrome or hypochondriasis. The paternal grandfather died of a brain tumor a year ago.

The stressors that could be identified were the party, her grandfather's death the previous year, and some conflict around the issue of independence. She described her parents as overprotective and sheltering, denied any psychological discomfort, and could not understand how her symptom could be anything but physically based. Her Minnesota Multiphasic Personality Inventory (MMPI) profile was within normal limits, with the exception of the Hypochrondriasis Scale, which was 2 standard deviations above the mean. Rorschach testing suggested a difficulty in expressing affect, preoccupation with somatic concerns, and conflict and stress interfering with her using her resources. The evaluation team detected no indications of severe psychopathology.

During the hospital stay, the team worked intensively with Kathy's parents, trying to help them understand their daughter's problem. They also told Kathy that her's was a psychological problem on which she needed to work. When she began to complain of pain in her leg, and her parents, who were cautioned not to ask her about it, did not, the leg pain disappeared. A program that included psychotherapy for both Kathy and her parents, with a simultaneous biofeedback program, was to be carried out in a county mental health clinic. Short-term follow-up indicates that Kathy's headaches have become less frequent.

Although Kathy had a long-standing series of somatic symptoms, they did not reflect any severe psychopathology at the time of her hospital stay. The progression from abdominal to headache pain may typify developing somatization disorders (Ernst, Routh, & Harper, 1984). Because Kathy's family perceived her as fragile, they infantilized her and ministered to her somatic symptoms. Her father was overly involved with her symptoms (a common finding in somatizing adolescent girls), and her mother did not modulate the potentially overstimulating closeness. The staff thought that Kathy's father's oversolicitous and perhaps somewhat seductive behavior exacerbated her symptoms, as did her mother's withdrawal. Kathy's parents were insightful enough to understand the formulation and agreed to work on changing these interactions. This type of somatoform disorder, in which the degree of psychopathology is relatively small, is probably the most common form in children, but the use of somatic symptoms as a coping strategy can become a lifelong adaptation if not discouraged.

Monosymptomatic Somatization Disorder (Type 2)

In a Type 2 disorder, the symptom is more than a language for the individual to express emotion, and it serves more than secondary gain. It expresses a continuous friction or stress involving the entire family. The symptom serves an important homeostatic function; everyone in the family needs it. Often, the symptom becomes the major focus of family discussions. By giving the family something on which to focus their energy, the symptom holds the family together in a common bond. Because the family depends on the symptom to maintain its precarious homeostasis, any precipitous attempt to remove it can persuade the family to transfer to another physician who will do more tests to establish that the symptom is a legitimate organic condition.

Alternatively, the symptom serves as a major coping mechanism to deal with the stress or conflict that precipitated somatization. For this type of situation to develop, several preconditions are usually necessary. First, since somatic symptoms are the focus of communication for the family, the family strongly reinforces the symptom. In addition, the child has a model in the family who uses somatic symptoms as a communication device, or who had an actual physical illness that elicited secondary gain. Finally, the child usually suffered a stressful precipitating event, often in the context of family strife. The likelihood that such a symptom will occur is higher in children with dependent or histrionic personalities.

Jessica is a 14-year-old girl admitted to the University of Minnesota Hospitals with severe pain in her right leg. No longer able to walk, she had not been attending school. Four months previously, a subcutaneous cyst had been removed from her leg. A few weeks after she recovered, the pain in her leg began again and made her limp. Since she was having trouble navigating the stairs at school, she felt she needed crutches and began using them. After winter vacation, she did not return to school, in part because she had begun to use a wheelchair.

Jessica's medical history revealed that she had had an ulcer at age 8. She had petit mal seizures diagnosed at age 5 and was treated with phenobarbitol until 4 years ago. She also has had migraine headaches treated with Cafergot. However, her only symptom at this admission was the leg pain.

Her social history revealed that Jessica's parents divorced when she was 8. She has not seen her biological father since then and feels that he does not like her as much as he likes her sister, and this feeling upsets her. History from the mother intimates that the biological father exposed himself to Jessica and abused the children physically, but neither the mother nor Jessica would state openly who his victims were.

Jessica's stepfather suffers from a bipolar affective disorder, is often out of control, and is on permanent disability, in part because of chronic low back pain. The stepfather is verbally and emotionally abusive, strict, and explosive. The mother, who suffers from systemic lupus erythematosus, behaves in a passive-aggressive manner. She often sides with the children against the stepfather. Jessica's sister has congenital kidney disease. A grandmother who lives in the household has congestive heart failure and is extremely obese, as are all the household members. Jessica is the thinnest member of the family.

Jessica says that her pain feels like someone is squeezing her leg from the knee down. To get relief she must stay in bed with her leg elevated, behavior that incidentally forces her sister to do all her chores and leaves her free to watch TV and do her homework. Although she says "I wish it would get better," she seems only minimally distressed. Affectively, she is pleasant but bland and seems mildly depressed when she talks about her symptom. No medicine relieves the pain; all treatments including baths and compresses and putting weight on her leg exacerbate it.

Jessica's parents are certain that their daughter is dreadfully ill and are solicitous to her because of her symptom. During Jessica's hospital stay, they persistently asked her about her physical symptoms, even after they were told that doing so was not in her best interest. She did not improve in the hospital and was discharged with a plan that included both biofeedback and psychotherapy, a plan that the parents reluctantly agreed to at first, and did not follow after Jessica was discharged.

Conversion Reaction of Childhood (Type 3)

Type 3 disorder is monosymptomatic, not necessarily more severe than Type 2, but qualitatively different. Most commonly, a clinician can identify a specific crisis or severe conflict that preceded the symptom. Often the child's life circumstances are conducive to somatic symptomatology because other ways to discharge emotion or resolve conflict or trauma are less available. A single physical symptom may develop that has some symbolic meaning for the subject and serves a pragmatic purpose. This may occur even in families without the characteristics noted above and in children who do not have a dependent or histrionic personality type.

In cases such as these, the child and the parents are less preoccupied with somatic illness, and psychotherapy or environmental manipulation may be most effective. These families usually are not reinforcing the symptoms or providing excessive secondary gain; in fact, the sudden onset of symptoms may perplex them. They often are amenable to the emotional and psychological explanation of the child's symptoms and, in contrast to families with other types of somatoform disorders, are often relieved that the child suffers from an emotional, not an organic, disease process. Generally, these children are not persistent somatizers. They conform more to the original Freudian concept of "conversion hysteria."

Lane is a 16-year-old boy whose parents brought him to the clinic. He had been unable to eat solid foods for the past several months because he was not able to swallow. The ear, nose, and throat and speech pathology services evaluated Lane and found no cause for his symptoms.

Lane had been followed in growth by the clinic since he was 5 because a pituitary injury at age 5 led to a growth failure. He has a slight left hemiparesis and some mild learning difficulties secondary to that accident. Prior to the onset of his current eating problems, Lane had contracted a virus, one of whose symptoms was a sore throat. His grandfather had died just prior to the onset of symptoms.

On interview, Lane was quiet, serious, and difficult to engage. He frequently became tearful, but he appeared to be unaware that he was crying. He described his mother as overly protective toward him, placing restrictions on his time with peers and opposing Lane's learning to drive. He wished his mother would give him more freedom and independence. Powerlessness and lack of ability to control events in his life, especially medical procedures and social interactions, were frequent themes.

On psychological tests, Lane was found to be of low average intelligence. Dysphoric themes were found on all his testing. Rorschach results indicated that Lane distanced himself from potential sources of distress. His protocol was consistent with depression, with a low number of responses, a low number of human responses, and an overall constricted picture. Stories on the Thematic Apperception Test were superficial and devoid of emotion. The MMPI indicated significant depression and paranoia, providing further corroboration that he felt helpless and unable to take charge of his life.

The evaluators concluded that Lane's conversion symptom was a response to his current feelings of helplessness, not wanting to "swallow" any more, and represented an effort to exert some control in his life. His conversion symptom also appeared to be secondary to a significant depressive episode.

Recommendations were for both individual psychotherapy and family sessions to help Lane take control of his life. In addition, biofeedback treatment to help Lane feel that he can control his body and gradually reintroduce other than soft foods to his diet was recommended. A description of his treatment can be found in Chapter 7.

Recent studies have found that some children develop conversion reactions in response to sexual molestation. The symptoms seem to be a strategy for coping with anxiety and overwhelming emotions resulting from severe external trauma, in addition to whatever preexisting familial stress might exist. Such symptom constellations are not strongly related to a particular type of personality disorder. The following short case report exemplifies the response to sexual trauma.

Sharon is a 14-year-old girl whose parents brought her to the hospital because she suddenly went blind following a seizure. Magnetic resonance and CT scans were negative. An ophthalmologic examination revealed variable visual acuity.

Sharon is a gifted child, who comes from a family in which she perceives much conflict that her parents are reluctant to discuss. Already considered a behavioral problem in the past year, she had been in psychiatric treatment. During her stay in the hospital, she reported that an acquaintance had raped her several weeks prior to the symptom's onset. She refused to identify the perpetrator. In addition, the stress of a new school, lack of seizure control, and interactional problems with her parents contributed to the development of this symptom.

Sharon was significantly depressed when she was first interviewed. She was discouraged about her symptoms, but despite insight into their cause, she did not demonstrate any motivation to overcome them. She maintained the symptom and an awareness of its cause simultaneously. Perhaps the strong oppositionality the evaluator noted contributed to the difficulty she had giving up the symptom. During her hospital stay, she stated that her blindness protected her from her other problems such as the rape. If she remained blind, she couldn't see what was going on in her life. The symptom also represented one way of getting attention and concern from her parents, who were somewhat distant and alienated from her.

Recommendations were for continued psychotherapy to deal with her feelings about the rape and biofeedback treatment to rid her of the symptom sufficiently to enable her to return to school. Because of her oppositionality, she may have needed a physical treatment like biofeedback to give up her symptom.

Somatization Disorder of Childhood (Type 4)

When family and physician reinforce and support specific symptoms, when multiple hospital admissions and laboratory investigations have been carried out, and when the stress within the family and the individual is high, the core symptoms begin to have other symptoms accreted onto them. An underlying personality disorder usually of a dependent or histrionic type, a high degree of stress, and the right combination of reinforcements are necessary to develop this polysymptomatic somatization syndrome. Usually, this combination of factors results in the symptoms becoming entrenched and the patient incapacitated. Chronic clusters of symptoms begin to emerge, similar to Briquet's syndrome in adults. Although relatively rare, such syndromes do occur in children. These children's parents infantilize them. They may do poorly in school, and sometimes even become bedridden. For this syndrome to develop, a child may need to have a severe preexisting personality disorder or an organic condition. Poor ego development and rigid defenses as well as a pathologic family environment are part of the clinical picture.

Anne is a 12-year-old girl who was admitted to the pediatric neurology service for a diagnostic evaluation to determine if her inability to talk, move her tongue, walk, and use her upper extremities was caused by neurologic or psychological forces. Anne had these symptoms for 10 months before she was hospitalized. The prior spring, she had returned home from a track meet fatigued, her eyes dilated, but with no other apparent illness and no evidence of ingested drug. She was hospitalized twice in her hometown, but no illness was found. After 2 weeks, she gradually began to lose her ability to talk normally and move her tongue and appeared to be progressively weaker. At the time of admission, Anne had some minor disuse atrophy of her upper arm muscles and had also become very demanding and controlling.

Anne had neuropsychological testing done soon after the onset of her illness. She was found to be of average intelligence, with difficulties in visual motor skills. This year she had been getting physical therapy, occupational therapy, speech therapy, and special education in school. Her parents had noted that she spoke normally on two occasions when she was surprised or angry. Two inpatient workups in major medical centers uncovered no neurologic impairment. She did not speak normally and looked as if she has cerebral palsy, although no neurologic abnormality had been found.

Anne was adopted when she was 6 weeks of age. Described by her parents as a "sweet" docile infant, she walked at 13 months and spoke and fed herself early. She had always been neat, well organized, prim, and somewhat immature. In special classes from second grade because of a learning disability, Anne had had special problems in math and difficulty completing homework. But she could always get other children to do her work for her. Her parents described her as moody, always wanting to be babied, and extremely difficult and demanding. She had been very worried about going to a new school next year. Anne was particularly upset about having to take showers after gym class. Last year, prior to the onset of symptoms, her parents noticed she was somewhat rebellious, refusing to do what they said. Following confrontations with her mother, Anne would often write her a long note saying how sorry she was. Since the symptoms began, these personality characteristics have been even more extreme. She has given up feeding and dressing herself, which she was previously perfectly able to do. Because her parents were fearful and guilty, they have been doing things for her, in this way reinforcing her dependency, symptomatology, and maladaptive behavioral patterns.

In an interview, Anne was reticent, communicating with difficulty and speaking only when questioned. Her passivity was effective in controlling others. She never spoke spontaneously, always waiting so that others would do things for her. She demonstrated no sadness or anger regarding her symptoms. Rorschach testing revealed that Anne was concerned about her own body and felt vulnerable. She was very suggestible and sensitive to the influence of her environment.

Because Anne's symptoms were so severe, the staff elected to try hypnosis initially. However, her symptoms were relieved only transiently. Noting that Anne's gait was much less impaired when she thought no one was observing her, the staff decided that Anne's problem was emotional and transferred her to the inpatient child psychiatry ward. When Anne was asked about her reaction to this transfer, she said she was self-conscious about the way she ate and was concerned that on the psychiatric ward she would have to eat in front of other people. She was also concerned that there was no one to help her get dressed. Even though Anne got others to tie her shoes for her, the staff observed that she was able to tie her own shoes after relaxation exercises if no help was offered.

The initial plan on the child psychiatry unit involved the removal of all secondary gain. However, hospitalization alone appeared to reinforce Anne's symptoms enough to keep them going. Thus, Anne had improved only mildly after a 3 month hospitalization. Her prognosis was guarded at best, and she was transferred to a residential treatment facility with the diagnosis of somatization disorder in a girl with a dependent personality. The cause of these extremely severe symptoms was never clarified.

These four subtypes of childhood somatoform disorders do not correspond clearly to the adult somatoform diagnoses listed in DSM III. The normal type, the nonspecific stress avoiders, are not dysfunctional and therefore do not fall into a diagnosable category. Normal adults also occasionally use somatic symptoms as stress avoiders.

Tentative criteria for diagnosis of these four types are shown below followed by a brief discussion of prognosis.

Type 1: Mild Polysymptomatic Somatization Disorder

1. History of persistent but nonspecific and changeable somatic symptoms, such as stomachaches, headaches, and malaise, with insidious onset over a period of several months.
2. History of physical illness in the patient or family members that serves as a model for secondary gain.

3. Symptoms primarily serve the purpose of secondary gain; parental reinforcement of dependency and focus on somatic symptoms are present.
4. Usually no other accompanying psychological symptoms.

TYPE 2: MONOSYMPTOMATIC SOMATIZATION DISORDER

1. Loss or alteration in physical functioning, suggesting a physical disorder, which is usually neurologic but can be gastrointestinal.
2. Acute onset with a temporally related stressor, usually familial.
3. History of physical illness in the patient or a close family member.
4. Symptoms serve the purpose of secondary gain, as well as stress reduction for both patient and family.
5. Often there are other accompanying psychological symptoms present, such as anxiety and depression.

TYPE 3: CONVERSION REACTION OF CHILDHOOD

1. Loss or alteration in physical functioning, suggesting a physical disorder, particularly a neurologic one.
2. Acute onset with a temporally related psychological stressor, usually but not solely related to sexual stress.
3. The symptom enables the patient to avoid a noxious activity.
4. No history of somatization or seeking secondary gain is necessary.

TYPE 4: SOMATIZATION DISORDER OF CHILDHOOD

1. History of various physical symptoms of more than 1 year's duration.
2. Complaints of at least five separate symptoms in any of the following categories; neurologic, gastrointestinal, pain, cardiopulmonary, and, in adolescent girls, gynecologic difficulties.
3. History of somatization in the patient and family members.
4. Often other psychological symptoms, such as anxiety and depression, accompany the disorder.

Children with a mild polysymptomatic somatization disorder (Type 1) show a mixed outcome. Some children develop somatization disorders as they grow up. Others are transient stress reactions with somatic symptomatology. It is very difficult to predict which children will fall into which category in the future. If the patient has more than one episode and the stressor he or she experiences does not seem very strong, it may be an early sign that a somatization disorder is developing. Kathy, described previously, may develop a somatization disorder since she had had seven prior hospitalizations for nonorganic symptoms. Other children with Type 1 dysfunction develop coping strategies that utilize less severe but persistent somatic symptoms, which help them avoid stress and anxiety, but which may never bring them to the attention of a psychologist or psychiatrist.

For the child with a monosymptomatic somatization disorder (Type 2), several outcomes are possible. Some children with such symptoms, especially those with deviant personality characteristics (such as histrionic or dependent behavior), have an incipient somatization disorder, which emerges with time and stress. For other children with more severe environmental stress, somatic symptomatology represents a cry for help. Jessica falls into this category. In some ways, she is the least disturbed member of her pathologic and emotionally abusive family. Since somatization is the family language, the somatic symptom is a ticket to help and attention. Although her current problem is primarily situational, whether she will develop significant psychopathology in the future remains to be seen.

The Type 3 disorder is similar to the adult conversion reaction. A precipitating event can be identified, which in some cases is sexual. In addition, the child's symptoms often take on a symbolic quality and communicate a message about the conflict. As in the adult disorder, both primary and secondary gain are present. The chaotic home milieu seen in somatization disorders is often absent. Psychotherapy and other interventions often result in good outcome, and several such children we have followed have remained symptom-free for several years.

Finally, the persistent somatization of the Type 4 disorder may be a childhood form of the adult somatization disorder. Our impression is that children with this disorder have a poor outcome. However, because such persistent, resistant, and well defined disorders are uncommon in childhood, we have limited outcome data.

As for other childhood disorders, DSM III does not always provide appropriate categories that account for developmental changes. In the case of somatoform disorders, DMS III criteria may be only partially applicable. Type 1 and 2 disorders appear to be unique to children, reflecting their developmental instability and their lack of formed psychopathology, vacillating between normality, adjustment reactions, and somatization disorders. Types 3 and 4 are early-appearing disorders that correspond to an adult conversion reaction and somatization disorder, respectively. However, even in the case of somatization disorder, because the child is young, the number of symptoms described in DSM III will not likely be present, nor will all the criteria for diagnosis be met. Thus, we feel that our criteria better reflect the manifestations of childhood disorders and the manifestations that help clinicians discriminate between them.

While we have elaborated the criteria for four categories of somatoform disorders, for research purposes it may be more prudent initially to classify children into monosymptomatic and polysymptomatic groups. To compare the characteristics of these two groups, we have studied 27 children with somatoform disorders and found differences in several areas, such as the presence of learning disabilities and family history of medical and somatoform illness in the polysymptomatic group (Shapiro & Rosenfeld, 1986). However, because of the great range of severity and the qualitative differences within the monosymptomatic and the polysymptomatic somatoform disorders, the categorization into four types may be more clinically useful for treatment decisions and prognostic considerations.

References

American Psychiatric Association. (1980). *Diagnostic and statistical manual of mental disorders* (3rd ed.). Washington, DC: Author.

Carek, D.J., & Santos, A.B. (1984). Atypical somatoform disorder following infection in children—a depressive equivalent? *Journal of Clinical Psychiatry, 45*, 108–111.

Ernst, A.R., Routh, D.K., & Harper, D. (1984). Abdominal pain in children and symptoms of somatization disorder. *Journal of Pediatric Psychology, 9*, 77–86.

Forbis, O.L., & Jones, R.H. (1965). Hysteria in childhood. *Southern Medical Journal, 58*, 1221–1225.

Goodyer, I. (1981). Hysterical conversion reactions in childhood. *Journal of Child Psychology and Psychiatry, 22*, 179–188.

Hinman, A. (1958). Conversion hysteria in childhood. *American Journal of Diseases in Children, 95*, 42–45.

Laybourne, T.C., & Churchill, S.W. (1972). Symptom discouragement in treating hysterical reactions in childhood. *International Journal of Psychotherapy, 1*, 111–123.

Looff, D.H. (1970). Psychophysiologic and conversion reactions in children. *Journal of the American Academy of Child Psychiatry, 9*, 318–331.

Maloney, M. (1980). Diagnosing hysterical conversion reactions in children. *Journal of Pediatrics, 97*, 1016–1020.

Proctor, J.T. (1958). Hysteria in childhood. *American Journal of Orthopsychiatry, 28*, 394–407.

Schneider, S., & Rice, D. (1979). Neurologic manifestations of childhood hysteria. *Pediatrics, 94*, 153–156.

Shapiro, E., & Rosenfeld, A.A (1986). Monosymptomatic and polysymptomatic somatoform disorders in children and adolescents. Unpublished manuscript.

Volkmar, F.R., Poll, J., & Lewis, M. (1984). Conversion reactions in childhood and adolescence. *Journal of the American Academy of Child Psychiatry, 23*, 424–430.

Whitlock, F.A. (1967). The aetiology of hysteria. *Acta Psychiatrica Scandinavica, 43*, 144–162.

Woodruff, R.A., Clayton, P.J., & Guze, S.B. (1969). Hysteria. *British Journal of Psychiatry, 128*, 1243–1248.

6

Principles of Diagnosis

Patients with somatoform symptoms usually first see pediatricians or general practitioners, not mental health professionals. Since many somatoform symptoms are initially indistinguishable from organic ones, the primary care physician must first make certain that the symptom is not part of a physical disease process.

However, approaching these patients with the attitude that their illness must be physical, doing a large battery of tests, and then concluding that since all the tests that could be done have turned up no organic findings, and the symptom must be psychological often results in the patient being dissatisfied and the physician frustrated. If an elaborate medical workup produces reams of negative results before the physician realizes that the illness is psychological, he or she can become annoyed with the patient for "pulling the wool over his or her eyes." This is less likely to happen if the physician considers the possibility that the symptom might be psychological when initiating the medical workup for an organic etiology. Knowing and applying specific criteria for somatoform disorders allow the primary care physician to be more confident in making a psychological diagnosis when it is appropriate. This permits better management and interventions specifically tailored to the child's diagnosis and needs.

In order to correctly identify the patient with a somatoform disorder, several crucial questions should be considered. (a) Is the symptom's onset related to any life event, personal loss, developmental crisis, or physical illness? Can such a correlation be objectively demonstrated? If no trigger is immediately apparent, what chronic conflict, stress, or covert problem could have precipitated the symptom? (b) Is there a history of neurologic disorder or family patterns that might indicate a predisposition to somatoform symptoms? (c) Is the family environment conducive to developing such symptoms? Does the family focus on somatic symptoms? Do other family members have somatic symptoms? Does anyone in the family have the same symptoms? How do the family members express their needs? Can they talk about their emotional responses? Do they have words for affects? Does the patient derive secondary gain from the symptom? (d) How does the child behave, and what are his or her personality traits? Are there indications of dependent or histrionic characteristics? (See Chapter 3 for

DSM III criteria.) What coping strategies or defense mechanisms does the child have in his or her repertoire? Have other, less dramatic defenses, been overwhelmed? Is the child indifferent to the symptom? Is *la belle indifférence* part of the presenting picture? (e) Does the peer environment also provide secondary gain or reinforcement of the symptoms?

Three components help assess these variables: an interview with the child, an interview with the parents (and perhaps the whole family), and a psychological evaluation of the child. In addition, reports from teachers and the school nurse can be invaluable aids in establishing a premorbid baseline. This diagnostic evaluation should be just that. Too often the physician, confusing diagnosis with treatment, intervenes too fast. The parents flee to another doctor seeking a cause for their child's symptom.

Although the following procedures are more likely to be carried out by a mental health professional, to a limited degree, some of these procedures should be part of the primary care physician's tools.

Interview with the Child

Obviously the interview format will depend on the age of the child. With children of normal intelligence who are 8 or older, a standard interview format can be adopted. Younger children will need more indirect ways of exploring their symptomatology, such as play interviews. With younger children, using dolls, puppets, or any other form of third person fantasy in which the child's symptoms can be ascribed to the imaginary characters often can help in exploring a symptom's meaning. Drawings, storytelling techniques, and role-playing can also be useful ways to ask direct concrete questions about symptomatology. "What happens if. . ." questions are particularly helpful. Examples are "What does the girl's mother do when she feels weak?" and "What will the girl do if her mother is not there?"

With preadolescent children, it is important to keep the questions concrete, oriented to "what" and not "why" questions (for example, asking "What happens when your headache gets worse?" or "What do your friends do when you are dizzy?" or "What does your mother do when you complain about your symptoms?"). "What" questions allow a child to describe his or her observations. "Why" questions about a child's behavior are intrusive rather than requests for objective information. They often make children defensive or make them feel accused. Also, the child may be cognitively unable to answer an etiologic question. General techniques for play interviews are addressed clearly by Simmons (1983).

Some recently developed structured interviews make useful suggestions about the general content of interviews. However, to our knowledge, the Diagnostic Interview Schedule for Children (DISC) (Costello, Edebrock, Kalas, Kessler, & Klarie, 1982) is the only one that has categories for both conversion and somatization disorder. The Diagnostic Interview for Children and Adolescents (Herjanic, 1981; Herjanic & Campbell, 1977) includes only somatization disorder. The Schedule for Affective Disorders and Schizophrenia for School Aged Children (Kiddie-SADS) (Puig-Antich & Chambers, 1978) has only affective and schizophrenic disorder categories. Although both are useful in delineating symptomatology frequently seen in mental health settings, they lack those items that would be helpful in a medical setting to diagnose somatoform disorders. Nevertheless, they are useful models for developing strategies for collecting interview data both from parents and children.

The most important part of the diagnostic interview is the exploration of the presenting symptoms. In the initial interview, the diagnostician should obtain a detailed description of the symptoms. With pain symptoms, the evaluation should discuss its quality, intensity, and location. Identifying circumstances that make the symptom better or worse is important. Are there associated complaints? What treatments have been tried and what effect have they had? The diurnal variation of the symptom is often significant. What has been the symptom's course? If more than one symptom is present, each should be explored separately.

The health care professional should pay attention to the small details of symptom presentation for several reasons. First, careful attention to detail helps the clinician to differentiate between organic and somatic complaints. Second, it may help him or her gain the trust of a patient who thinks that others are not taking the symptoms seriously enough. A professional who respects a patient's symptoms will often gain the patient's respect in return. Developing trust around this issue is very important since if the workup uncovers no organic pathology, the clinician may have to explain a complex psychological etiology. If the patient and parents feel that the clinician appreciated the symptom and explored it in depth rather than shrugged it off without careful attention, they will be more likely to accept whatever recommendations he or she makes for treatment.

The clinician should explore in detail the context in which the symptom first appeared since important information as to the precipitating stressor for the somatoform symptom is often unknowingly disclosed during this description. Throughout the interview, the examiner should be aware that because the conflict and causes of the symptom are outside the patient's conscious awareness, much of what he or she is looking for is inferential. Thus, phenomena during the interview, such as sudden shifts of affect, changes in the flow of verbalization, changing of the subject, slips of the tongue, changes in eye contact, and other signs that might be indicative of anxiety or avoiding anxiety-laden topics, should be attended to carefully and recorded as clues that may help detect the noxious stimulus that the symptom helps the patient avoid.

Another important area to explore is the effect of the child's environment on the symptoms. The role of parental, sibling, and peer reaction in making the symptoms better or worse and in perpetuating them needs to be identified. Conditions that increase the secondary gain and keep the conflict level low are important factors in maintaining the symptom and should be explored. Careful attention to the symptom's response to the diagnostic process can often give the diagnostician clues to the best intervention strategy. Children who somatize often respond positively to hospitals and doctors. These children, who may have a symptom such as persistent headaches or a leg paralysis, have no attacks while in the hospital. However, immediately after discharge, they are back in the clinic with severe symptoms. This seems to indicate that something in the home environment is exacerbating their condition. If the inpatient diagnostic process is not handled appropriately, it may contribute to a symptom's perpetuation because the only way the child can avoid being home is to remain ill. In some cases, the home environment will need to be altered substantially before the child can live there comfortably.

The child's attitude to his or her ailment is also important to explore. The child with a somatoform disorder often has an inappropriate affective response to the symptoms. Although these inappropriate affects range from overdramatization to total lack of anxiety or worry, the latter most commonly characterizes the conversion reaction. Children with histrionic personality patterns will often seem to be very concerned, almost "hysterical" (in the lay sense) about their symptoms, but often this affective response is shallow and attention-seeking. On the other hand, unconcern with gross debility, or *la belle indifférence* is a fairly common finding associated with conversion symptoms, especially in children with dependent or more normal personality configurations.

In addition, the evaluation ought to explore the cognitions (ideas and thoughts), fantasies, and beliefs the patient has about the symptoms. Where do such symptoms come from? What might make them go away? Does anyone else know you have such symptoms? Did anything they or you did influence your symptoms? Do your symptoms make you feel differently about yourself? If the patient believes he or she is incurable, is being punished for misdeeds by God, has a hereditary disorder, will only be taken care of if severely ill, or has any other mistaken belief, these beliefs should not be attacked. They must be gradually altered before symptom relief can be obtained. The child should be encouraged to incorporate alternative coping strategies that will result in the gradual diminution and disappearance of the symptom. Direct suggestion and environmental manipulation of secondary gain are appropriate therapeutic interventions that will be discussed later.

In addition to the detailed investigation of symptoms, a more general interview format is also recommended to explore questions about family interactions, and the child's social and academic environment. How affect is expressed in these contexts and how stress is handled are particularly important. Children with chronic somatoform reactions have only a few strategies to help them meet their needs; their coping mechanisms are ineffective in handling stress and conflict. They have few rational and intellectual strategies available due, in part, to their verbal inability to express affect and to their lack of psychological-mindedness. They utilize repression and denial as their sole defense mechanisms. Some children of high ability and/or greater insight generally may try out conversion symptoms as a coping strategy, but will abandon them more quickly, realizing that these strategies are both ineffective and counterproductive to general growth and development.

Thus, the interview with the child may help to make the diagnosis of somatoform disorder clear. However, in many milder cases of somatization, the patient seems to be functioning well psychologically. Outside of the specific symptomatology, the patient suffers no overt anxiety, shows no undue concern about the symptom, and does not act out or seem depressed. The patient is usually pleasant, eager to talk about his or her symptomatology, and frequently shows little affect. Since many health professionals consider somatization a bit devious and manipulative, patients who seem like nice everyday people are more likely to be considered people with an unfortunate but obscure medical condition. In such cases, even physicians who consider the possibility of somatization in their differential diagnosis may fail to make the diagnosis because the psychopathology is hard to detect. Such conversion reactions have fooled many competent psychologists and psychiatrists. Furthermore, because pediatricians and general practitioners see most of these cases and usually do not refer them for psychological or psychiatric evaluation, many mental health professionals have had little exposure to such patients.

Interview with the Parents

A thorough assessment of the family environment, including careful attention to the parents' description of the child's symptomatology, is crucial in evaluating any child suspected of having somatoform symptoms. As with the child interview, the evaluation should thoroughly examine the symptom complex from the parents' viewpoint.

This helps to build trust between the parents and the clinician. By discussing various facets of the symptoms carefully and systematically, the clinician demonstrates to the parents that he or she takes the symptoms seriously and considers them legitimate, not figments of their child's or their own imagination. It is important to avoid being condescending or disbelieving to the parents or seeming to doubt their story. In addition, one should assess how difficult it might be for them to understand and accept a psychological view of their child's disorder.

The psychiatrist or psychologist should strive to establish an alliance with the family as a clinician interested in the psychological aspects of the symptoms who is working with physicians who are investigating the physical basis of the disorder. Often, when the parents realize that their fears are being taken seriously, they can be less defensive; many become more flexible once trust is established. Many of these families need to be managed patiently.

Once again, the parental interview must carefully assess the symptom's onset. It may be worthwhile to encourage psychologically naive parents to describe in detail everything that was happening at the time of the symptom began without asking them to associate those events to the symptom. In addition, the patient's premorbid personality, any changes in behavior that may have occurred, and a detailed account of all interventions that have been attempted and their outcome should be obtained.

While listening to the parent's description of what interventions have been attempted, the clinician should evaluate whatever secondary gain the parents offer the patient for the symptoms. Parents should be encouraged to describe whether their behavior toward the patient has changed, and how the patient's symptoms have affected the family's functioning. The description will often clarify what interest and emotional investment the parents have in the child's symptoms. What meaning does this symptom have for the parents? Exploring parental medical histories, especially whether they have experienced the same symptoms in the past or currently, and their own tendencies to focus on somatic complaints will allow the interviewer to assess the extent to which the parents identify with the child's symptoms.

Parents can be asked what hypotheses they have had about the etiology of their child's symptoms. Do they think psychological stressors caused the symptoms, or do they consider the symptoms to be reflections of serious organic illness? The answer to this may be helpful in perceiving the parents' view of the disorder and their receptivity to psychological explanation or intervention.

Many families in which somatization is an important family style resist and even resent the idea that psychological factors may play a role in their child's symptoms. In fact, parents whose children have somatoform symptoms will refuse to let a psychologist or psychiatrist be involved in the child's care because they are convinced the illness is entirely organic. This objection can often be circumvented if the pediatrician suggests that the psychiatric or psychological examination is a routine but important part of every medical workup for those physical symptoms that might be exacerbated by stress.

Another problem is that some patients with somatoform disorders are not psychologically-minded. Such patients lack the ability to understand psychological mechanisms and to describe emotions in themselves or others. This makes it more difficult to communicate effectively with them and to collect important historic data.

The evaluator should determine whether family members' needs get satisfied through the somatic symptoms and whether family members have coping strategies other than somatization. The expression of affects within the family can be assessed both by direct questions and by observing the interaction among family members.

Because assessing family dynamics and interpersonal relationships is important, a family interview is recommended at some point in the diagnostic process. Family members' attitudes and behavior toward the identified patient will help to clarify whether the symptom is a means of resolving conflict or distress among family members. The stresses and conflicts impinging on family members other than the identified patient may be important. Job difficulties, marital conflicts, impending changes and separations, deaths, and illnesses all may be contributing factors in upsetting the family's homeostasis. If no ways of communicating and expressing affect other than somatization are available, somatic symptoms may emerge in the family member currently most stressed or in another "willing" to accept the role of the sick one to be worried about (e.g., a child becomes symptomatic and his fighting parents stop arguing and begin to work together to help him).

The evaluator should ask the parents what the patient has done to deal with stress in the past. The questions the parents are asked should be chosen to reveal the way the parents see the child's personality. The evaluator should discuss the child's social development, general temperament, behavioral characteristics, anxiety level, sexual development, and how he or she expresses feelings. In addition, cognitive assets and deficits as well as cognitive style and defense mechanisms should be explored. One way to do this is to discuss a situation that the evaluator or parents know stressed the child. The event could be the birth of a new sibling, the death of a relative, or parental divorce, for example. Ask questions such as How did Tommy express his feelings about this event? How did it affect his mood? his school work? His sociability? Does he express feelings openly? If so, how? If not, did keeping them bottled up affect him? Did he get physically sick? How do you know when he is anxious, unhappy, angry, frustrated? When things don't go well, how does he respond? Whom does he blame? Clearly, the evaluator will be especially interested in what types of somatic symptoms the patient has previously complained of, including those with a substantiated organic basis.

This information is best gathered with each parent interviewed separately. This allows each of them to express concerns and characteristic modes of coping that may not be obvious or that one of them might not feel free to share in a joint interview. Parents must understand that asking "psychological" questions is part of a routine workup, and does not imply that the symptoms are "imaginary."

Psychological Evaluation

The psychological evaluation is the third important dimension of the diagnostic workup. Although these tests cannot substitute for the interview with the child and the family, psychological tests can help make a diagnosis. Projective tests and the MMPI can help illuminate psychodynamics, personality characteristics, and the resources available to the patient. In addition, tests of intelligence and other cognitive and neuropsychological functions can identify limitations and assets in the child's repertoire that may have a bearing on personality diagnosis and treatment recommendations.

Since each child presents specific problems that may require quite different assessment approaches, a routine battery of tests cannot be recommended. But some basic tests with general clinical usefulness have been shown to identify characteristics specific to somatoform disorders. We will describe those tests and discuss some of our findings. However, the results we report in this section come from studies of children referred to a pediatric neurology clinic and, thus, may represent only one particular subset of children with somatoform disorders.

Cognitive Assessment

About two-thirds of the children with somatoform symptoms we have evaluated have had concomitant learning difficulties. Standard psychological tests have a limited ability to detect subtle residuals of early developmental deficits that parents describe. Compensatory strategies that accompany maturation during late childhood and adolescence mask them. This is particularly the case with language and visual motor functions. Thus, gathering historic information, searching for subtle residual deficits, and using (and developing) tests to measure these more subtle disabilities constitute the main objective of the neuropsychological evaluation.

Although the Wechsler Intelligence Scale for Children-Revised (WISC-R) is not very sensitive to such residuals of developmental deficit, it gives important information about the child's perceptual and cognitive style that may affect his or her personality configuration. It may also shed light on underlying cognitive patterns that may reflect the neurologic organization that predisposes the child to somatoform disorder. The most universal finding among children referred to the pediatric neurology clinic with somatoform disorders is the inability to perform arithmetic calculations. Figure 6.1 compares 10 children with somatoform disorders with 7 children with migraine or tension headache on WISC-R subtest scores. Each subject's subtest score was subtracted from his or her own mean score, and the deviation from the subjects own mean was calculated (a method proposed by Kaufman [1979]). The deviation score of -2.7 is significant at the $p = .01$ level.

The cause of poor arithmetic capability in children with somatoform disorder is unclear, but in every case that we evaluated, the score on the Arithmetic sub-

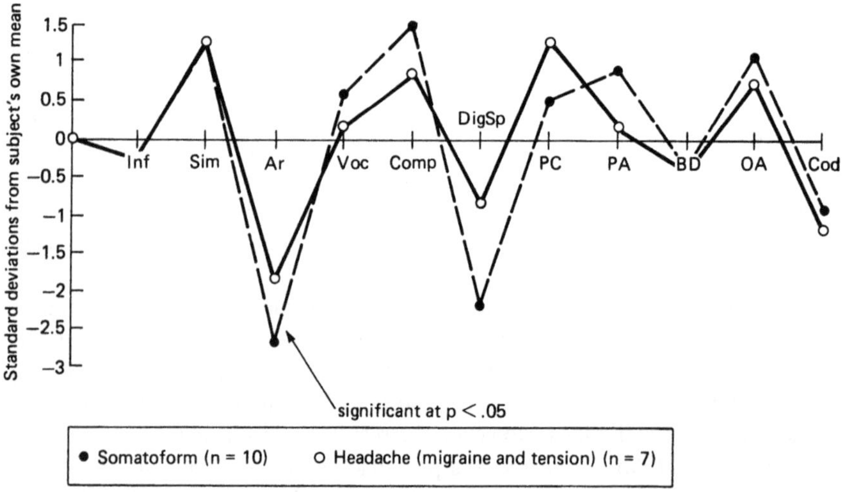

FIGURE 6.1. Mean deviation scores for WISC-R subtests.

test on the WISC-R is low relative to the rest of the profile. Several theories may explain these findings. It is important to note that mathematics may require more interhemispheric transfer of information than any other subtest. In this complex task, both left hemisphere verbal processing and right hemisphere spatial reasoning and focused attention are required. Thus, adequate communication between the hemispheres is crucial to good performance in mathematic reasoning. This observation is intriguing since an interhemispheric transfer problem is also consistent with the hypothesis that a disconnection between the left and right hemispheres contributes to difficulties in processing affective information in these children (see Chapter 3).

Because the Arithmetic subtest measures mental calculation, one may hypothesize that inattentiveness and impulsivity might be factors that contribute to these children's poor performance. This is consistent with research findings of selective inattention in adults with somatoform disorders (see Chapter 3). Psychologists giving the Wechsler tests to children with somatoform symptoms do, in fact, describe their behavior on cognitive testing as impulsive, inattentive to detail, and compliant with little performance anxiety. Some children with somatoform disorders show general difficulty with the freedom from distractibility subtests (Coding, Digit Span, and Arithmetic). Performance on other tests of attention, such as the Continuous Performance Test, is variable, but some children have great difficulty inhibiting responses on this test when the stimulus is presented frequently (errors of commission).

Other plausible explanations for poor mathematics ability are a deficit in spatial reasoning and problems in mental control as reflected in frontal lobe dysfunction. However, other test results do not support the hypothesis of consistent deficits in these areas.

Children with somatoform symptoms characteristically score well in several areas. Relative to their other scores, they have good scores on the Comprehension, Similarities, and Picture Arrangement subtests of the Wechsler scales. Such children are very aware of social reinforcements and social cues; they always seek interpersonal approval. Their knowledge of social conventions is well developed, and they perform nicely on tests that have social content.

The presence of right or left hemisphere dysfunction is not reflected in the WISC-R profiles of such children. Our WISC-R findings do not support those that hypothesize subtle left hemisphere language dysfunction and resultant right hemisphere predominance. Two points must be kept in mind in assessing our impressions. First, adults and children have been found to lateralize symptoms differently. Thus, the type of left hemisphere findings that have been observed in adults may not yet have consolidated in these children. Second, the WISC-R is not sensitive to subtle language dysfunction and, thus, may not illustrate subtle difficulties even if present. Even though their test scores fall in the normal range, many of these children do demonstrate imprecision and lack of syntactic organization in their language.

Other characteristics of some children with somatoform disorders, such as lack of vigilance and field dependence, are sometimes reflected in WISC-R performance. Children who employ repression and denial as coping strategies show patterns that include low scores on Picture Completion, Picture Arrangement, and sometimes Block Design.

Visual motor tests rarely reveal any errors of a blatantly organic type. Tests that we use are the Bender Gestalt, the Beery Developmental Test of Visual Motor Integration, and the Rey Osterreith. Performance is usually in the low average range. However, we have noted a lack of attention to small detail, imprecision, and sometimes poor organization. Some children with somatoform symptoms were reported by parents to have had slow motor development and, in their early years, had poor performance on visual motor tests according to school psychologist reports. Since we usually see these patients in late childhood and early adolescence, all but the most dysfunctional have made visual motor compensations.

These children's performance on most other tests of cognition, language, information processing, memory, and attention is usually within the average range. A characteristic lack of exactness, imprecision in language, and mild inattentiveness may be present. Although school performance may be poor, low normal or normal scores on individually administered achievement batteries may be found with the exception of mathematics, which is frequently deficient. Although many children with somatoform disorders have had special education for learning disabilities, by the time we see them their dysfunction is minimal (with the exception of mathematics). In our experience, most neuropsychological batteries, such as the Luria Nebraska Neuropsychological Battery or the Halstead Reitan Neuropsychological Battery, lack the sensitivity to detect the mild dysfunctions that are present in these patients because their scores are usually in the normal range.

Personality Assessment

Results of objective personality tests in these children are usually characterized by being "overnormal." They deny psychological symptomatology. On self-report measures of anxiety and depression (e.g., the Children's Manifest Anxiety Scale or Child Depression Inventory), usually only one or two items are endorsed other than the ones that reflect somatic symptomatology. The Minnesota Multiple Personality Inventory (MMPI) usually reflects a similar pattern. Although a substantial number of cases show elevations on scales 1 and 3 (Hypochondriasis and Hysteria) as well as *K* (test-taking attitude of defensiveness), these account for only about one-third of the total. Many profiles have very low scores on scales 2 and 7 (Depression and Psychasthenia). In fact, about one-third of the profiles may be within normal limits since the patient is not reporting psychological distress. However, for a significant number of children who have somatic symptoms where the symptom is not relieving the stress or conflict, one may find any number of patterns. Depression may be elevated, or *PD* (Psychopathic

Deviate) is elevated if the patient is acting out. More severe psychopathology is reflected by elevations on *F* and Schizophrenia usually associated with multiple symptomatology.

Projective tests may indicate the degree of distress and anxiety the patient experiences, how oriented to reality the child is, and the degree of the child's somatic preoccupation. Generally, we treat projective data as additional information to add to the diagnostic picture and do not use it for diagnostic purposes. The role of projective tests is as an adjunct; they are not useful in making diagnoses in isolation. But the Rorschach test, in particular, can yield important information about cognitive and perceptual style.

We have collected the Rorschach protocols of 14 children of average intelligence, between the ages of 8 and 16 years, who were identified as having a somatoform disorder in the pediatric neuropsychology clinic of the Division of Pediatric Neurology at the University of Minnesota (Table 6.1). These children were divided into two groups: monosymptomatic or polysymptomatic. The monosymptomatic group (MS) met either the criteria for conversion reaction or monosymptomatic somatization disorder as defined in Chapter 5. The polysymptomatic group (PS) included children who met the mild polysymptomatic somatization disorder or somatization disorder criteria.

These are cases where the protocols were administered, scored, and recorded using Exner's Comprehensive System (Exner, 1974). For several summary variables, scores were transformed into *Z* scores using normative scores for the subject's age to make them comparable across ages. For each variable in the Exner system, if the average *Z* score was more than 1.5, it was considered significant.

Nine children (eight females and one male) comprised the MS group. The PS group included four females and one male. No differences in mean age for the two groups was found. Twelve of the 14 had prior neurologic and medical problems, and 9 of the 14 had a prior history of learning disability. All of the PS group had other psychological symptoms (anxiety, depression, etc.), and two of the five had sexual concerns. Five of the nine MS children had psychological symptoms, and four of the seven had sexual concerns. These data are summarized in Table 6.2.

The most dramatic finding was the difficulty in perceptual accuracy in children with somatoform disorders. All the significant deviations from age norms reflect poor ability to respond as other children do to the configuration of the inkblots (Table 6.3). Of the 14 children in the sample, only 2 had a normal *F*+ % or *X*+ % (measures of how well the percept fits the inkblot, as determined by frequencies in the normal population). There was also a large number of unusual detail (*Dd*) responses. Adding to this picture of poor reality testing is the high number of special scorings (use of unusual language, reasoning, or content in describing percepts such as deviant verbalizations, alogical reasoning, contaminations, etc.) in the entire group of 14 children. Unusual locations, faulty reasoning, and the high schizophrenia index are consistent with the work of Flor-Henry, Fromm-Auch, Tapper, and Schopflocher (1981), in which neuropsychological similarities between somatoform disorders and schizophrenia in adults were found.

TABLE 6.1. Characteristics of Sample Given Rorshach Tests

Patient	Age	Presenting Symptoms	Prior Medical Problems	Learning Disabilities	Psychological Problems
Polysymptomatic Group[a]					
Laura[b]	11.0	Seizures, falling, leg weakness	Migraine, left ataxia, leg weakness	Mild	Fearful, hystrionic, sexual concerns
Kathy[b]	14.10	Severe headaches, multiple complaints	Reye syndrome, migraine	None	Dependency, repression
Jessica[c]	15.8	Leg pain, unable to walk, multiple complaints	Epilepsy, migraine, leg cyst	Moderate	Anxiety, depression, sexual concerns
Carol[c]	13.8	Unable to walk, pain in legs	Headaches, multiple illnesses	Moderate	Anxiety, dysphoria, bizarre thoughts
David[c]	13.11	Pseudoseizures, dizzyness, blind spells	Epilepsy/partial complex	Severe	Passive aggressive, mild depression
Monosymptomatic Group[d]					
Donna[e]	10.1	Hearing loss, tinnitus	Migraine	None	Immaturity, anxiety
Lisa[e]	15.0	Headache, neck-pain	Focal retinitis	Mild	Anxiety, withdrawal
Sandra[e]	9.8	Pain, weakness in legs	Infection in one leg	Mild	Fearful, dependent, sexual concerns
Mary[f]	14.8	Paralysis of right hand	None	Mild	Separation anxiety, sexual concerns
Cheryl[f]	14.6	Fainting, headaches	None	None	Dependency, fear of sexuality
Judy[f]	15.7	Muscle jerking, tinnitus	Absence epilepsy	None	Mild avoidance of affect
Tammy[f]	12.5	Pseudoseizures	Febrile seizures	Mild	Sexual concerns
Missy[e]	16.1	Dystonia of the tongue	Ovarian cysts, surgical complications	None	Avoidance of negative affect
Andy[e]	16.0	Dysphagia	Pituitary injury, left hemiparesis	Moderate	Depression, excessive passivity

[a] Mean age 13 years, 8 months.
[b] Mild polysymptomatic somatization disorder.
[c] Polysymptomatic somatization disorder.
[d] Mean age 13 years, 9 months.
[e] Monosymptomatic somatization disorder.
[f] Conversion disorder.

TABLE 6.2. Rorshach Scores of Children with Somatoform Disorders

	Rorschach Score																
Patient	*R*	*W*	*D*	*Dd*	*S*	*M*	*FM*	*m*	*FC*	*CF*+ *C*	Total Shading	*FD*	*Prs*	*F*	Blends	*P*	*Z*	*Zd*
Polysymptomatic Group																		
Laura	32	10	15	7	2	2	4	2	3	3	1	0	11	14	4	5	11	−8.5
Kathy	31	4	13	15	1	2	4	0	0	0	1	0	4	20	4	4	6	0
Jessica	30	17	8	5	3	6	2	0	1	0	0	0	9	20	1	8	17	−4.5
Carol	64	3	34	27	8	1	0	0	2	2	6	0	9	46	1	7	5	−0.5
David	13	7	4	2	0	3	3	0	2	0	1	1	4	4	0	5	8	6.5
Group mean	34.00	8.20	14.80	11.20	2.80	2.80	2.60	0.40	1.60	1.00	1.80	0.20	7.40	20.80	2.00	5.80	9.40	−1.40
Monosymptomatic Group																		
Donna	16	10	5	1	0	5	1	0	0	0	1	0	11	5	4	6	11	1
Lisa	9	5	1	3	3	1	1	0	1	0	0	0	1	6	0	3	5	−0.5
Sandra	15	7	3	5	1	3	0	0	0	0	1	1	9	2	8	7	12	2.5
Mary	30	13	9	8	2	7	1	1	0	0	4	1	8	7	9	10	23	−8
Cheryl	22	14	7	1	2	2	3	0	3	1	0	0	2	10	1	5	15	−6.5
Judy	24	10	14	0	0	4	2	0	2	0	4	0	14	7	5	8	13	
Tammy	11	9	1	1	0	1	2	0	1	0	0	0	5	6	1	5	10	2.5
Missy	11	2	6	3	1	1	0	0	0	0	1	0	7	8	1	6	4	−4
Andy	20	6	9	5	4	0	1	1	1	0	2	0	3	13	1	3	6	0
Group mean	17.56	8.44	6.11	3.00	1.44	2.67	1.22	0.22	0.89	0.11	1.44	0.22	6.67	7.11	3.33	5.89	11.00	−1.63
Total group mean	23.43	8.36	9.21	5.93	1.93	2.71	1.71	0.29	1.14	0.43	1.57	0.21	6.93	12.00	2.86	5.86	10.43	−1.54
12 year norms	20.6	7.2	11.7	1.7	0.9	3.1	3.6	0.4	2	2.7	2.1	0.8	8.8	8.7	3.9	6.1	9.5	−0.3

TABLE 6.2. *Continued*

	Rorschach Score															
	F+	*X*+	Σ*M*	Σ*C*	*EA*	Σ *FM*+ *m*	Σ *Shad*	*es*	Lambda	El	Aff Ratio	H	*A*	Spec Score	Dep Index	Scz Index
Polysymptomatic Group																
Laura	0.4	0.3	2	6.5	8.5	9	2	11	0.77	0.34	113	3	0.63	11	3	3
Kathy	0.6	0.6	3	1	2	5	3	8	1.8	0.32	55	2	0.66	1	0	1
Jessica	0.3	0.4	6	0.5	6.5	3	0	3	2	0.3	33	9	0.5	8	1	4
Carol	0.6	0.6	2	3.5	5.5	0	12	12	2.6	0.14	35	4	0.36	14	2	4
David	0.5	0.5	3	1	4	3	0	3	0.44	0.77	63	3	0.46	3	0	2
Group mean	0.47	0.48	3.20	2.50	5.30	4.00	3.40	7.40	1.52	0.37	59.80	4.20	0.52	7.40	1.20	2.80
Monosymptomatic Group																
Donna	0.6	0.6	8	2.5	10.5	4	1	5	0.45	0.68	45	10	0.3	2	0	1
Lisa	0.7	0.4	1	0.5	1.5	1	0	1	2	0.11	29	1	0.55	0	1	2
Sandra	0.5	0.4	6	6.5	12.5	4	9	13	0.15	0.6	25	9	0.2	13	3	2
Mary	0.3	0.4	12	2.5	14.5	9	12	21	0.23	0.27	40	11	0.43	7	2	4
Cheryl	0.5	0.4	3	3	6	3	0	3	0.83	0.36	29	0	0.68	7	0	3
Judy	1	0.8	6	3	9	4	7	11	0.41	0.58	118	5	0.67	0	1	0
Tammy	0.8	0.7	2	1	3	2	0	2	1.2	0.45	36	5	0.45	1	0	2
Missy	1	1	1	1	1.5	1	1	2	2.7	0.64	38	2	0.55	0		
Andy	0.5	0.5	0	0.5	0.5	2	3	5	1.86	0.15	43	1	0.4	1		
Group mean	0.66	0.59	4.33	2.28	6.56	3.33	3.67	7.00	1.09	0.43	44.78	4.89	0.47	3.44	1.00	2.00
Total group mean	0.59	0.55	3.93	2.36	6.11	3.57	3.57	7.14	1.25	0.41	50.14	4.64	0.49	4.86	1.08	2.33
12 year norms	0.8	0.8							0.73	0.47	0.73	2.4	0.43			

TABLE 6.3. Significant Deviations Expressed in Z Scores for Rorshach Variables for the Two Somatoform Groups

Name	*R*-M/S.D.[a]	*Dd*-M/S.D.	*F*+%-M/S.D.	*X*+%-M/S.D.	Lambda-M/S.D.	*Afr*-M/S.D.	*H*-M/S.D.
Polysymptomatic group							
Laura	2.88	6.5	−4.56	−4.82	−0.52	2.80	0.27
Kathy	1.76	14.67	−1.83	−2.11	9.18	−1.18	−0.44
Jessica	1.48	3.63	−4.67	−4.56	8.36	−2.44	3.94
Carol	8.31	22.64	−2.27	−3.00	10.76	−4.11	1.20
David	−1.69	−0.09	−2.91	−3.11	−1.94	−1.00	0.20
Mean score	2.55	9.47	−3.25	−3.52	5.17	−1.19	1.03
				MAbs	6.15		
Monosymptomatic group							
Donna	−0.95	−0.83	−1.90	−2.00	−2.25	−2.43	4.73
Lisa	−2.31	1.33	−1.25	−4.11	11.00	−2.71	−1.56
Sandra	−1.18	5.83	−3.30	−4.67	−4.13	−3.86	4.07
Mary	1.57	6.89	−4.42	−4.22	−5.09	−1.76	9.56
Cheryl	0.09	−0.89	−2.67	−4.44	0.36	−2.71	−2.67
Judy	0.33	−2.63	1.42	0.22	−3.00	2.88	1.44
Tammy	−2.00	−0.57	−0.45	−0.83	1.94	−2.33	2.09
Missy	−2.17	1.13	1.42	2.11	13.36	−2.13	−1.56
Andy	−0.44	3.63	−2.42	−4.00	7.36	−1.81	−0.44
Mean score	−0.79	1.54	−1.51	−2.44	2.17	−1.87	1.74
				MAbs	5.39		

[a] Actual score minus the mean score for age/standard deviation for age.
[b] Mean of the absolute values.

There was a group of normal scores for both groups. The number of popular responses, for example, was normal in both, as was the egocentricity index (a measure which indicates the degree of self-esteem; low scores are seen in depressed individuals). Human responses were high, reflecting the need for social approval that children with somatoform disorders have. *M* (human movement; a reflection of inner life or fantasy) responses were within the normal range. Consistent with this is the low depression index and the general lack of indicators of anxiety and distress, such as shading, vista, and achromatic color responses. In fact, the lack of experienced discomfort extends to a general lack of psychological-mindedness, as reflected in few vista responses.

The PS group gave large numbers of responses to the protocol, and accordingly, a large number of concrete details and form only responses. Lower *Z* scores (organization), high Lambda (ratio of form only responses to responses that have other determinants; higher numbers reflects more constriction), and Affective Ratio (ratio of responses to achromatic inkblots to responses to chromatic inkblots, usually indicating the degree of sensitivity to emotional stimuli) reflect a constricted, concrete, unambitious approach to the test in the PS group.

In contrast, the MS group had a more normal number of responses, a more organized, and a somewhat more elaborated style. The children in the MS group had more resources at their disposal (as indicated by the *EA* score) than did the

PS group. However, they were still below the expectable level in measures of perceptual accuracy and reality testing. An interesting finding was that their $F+\%$ (form quality of form only responses) was higher than their $X+\%$ (form quality of all responses), suggesting that for this group, emotional stimuli interfere with perceptual accuracy. The difficulty these children have expressing themselves appropriately around affective matters is also reflected in incongruous combinations in integrating color and form.

In general, the PS group had more unusual Rorschach protocols and deviant scores. Perhaps the multiple symptomatology is associated with more neurologic vulnerability and generally more psychological disturbance. Such patients may have an insidious personality disorder since a specific environmental stressor is not usually found in the PS syndrome. In contrast, the MS syndrome may be an adaptation to stress with few familial or endogenous factors.

It must be stressed that these results cannot be generalized since this is a pilot study on a small sample. These are children in a tertiary care center and are not randomly selected.

Responses to the Thematic Apperception Test have been less helpful in establishing the diagnosis, but quite useful in identifying the dynamics or conflicted impulses in the patient. Repeated themes, repeated omissions, storytelling style, outcomes, use of various defensive or coping strategies, description of affective response, and the intensity of affects in the stories may all contribute to the evaluator's understanding of the symptom's role in relieving stress.

One other useful technique in assessing children with somatic symptoms is to have them draw a human figure with the body part with the symptom and ask them to illustrate how the symptom feels. It sometimes helps to ask them to draw what they think is wrong with their body. Sentence completions, story completions, and family drawings are additional techniques that may be helpful.

Sexual Abuse and the Diagnostic Evaluation

Certain types of symptom presentations have more sexual overtones and are associated more frequently with sexual concerns. Pseudoseizures, leg paralyses, loss of consciousness, and those symptoms that are especially sudden in onset may be related to a prior sexual assault. In these cases, the patient may ultimately reveal these incidents. By law in many states, the professional must report any suspicion of sexual abuse to the proper authorities. Obviously, if a parent is the alleged perpetrator, this reporting creates a crisis that makes it quite difficult to continue a diagnostic evaluation. If the father is the perpetrator, he may end up going to jail, the child victim may be temporarily removed from the home, and this breakup of the home may result in a complete reshuffling of the professionals involved.

On the other hand, if the diagnostic evaluation continues, particularly when an outsider has molested the child, airing the incident and dealing with its emotional and social sequelae may be an important step toward resolving the symptoms.

More commonly, the clinician may suspect a sexual precipitant such as abuse, but the patient is not willing to share that information, or if the patient shares it, he or she retracts the accusation quickly. The patient can be reticent for several reasons. First, if the incident involves a family member, natural allegiance intervenes, as does a great deal of ambivalence towards that family member. The child may want the abuse to end if it is ongoing, but cannot bear the guilt of revealing the crime. Second, the child is ashamed and/or feels responsible for the crime. Children who somatize may tend to view everything in black and white terms and have a strong motivation always to be "good." Thus, children who have been sexually abused may see themselves as bad and guilty even if the sexual activity was forced upon them. This may serve an important defensive function for the child, as Wasserman and Rosenfeld (1985) have pointed out. If the actions of the abuser are the result of the child's bad behavior, then if the child can change his or her behavior and become good, all will be well. However, if the child believes his or her parent, who is the most important person in the world to a young child, is simply a bad person, life is utterly hopeless and the child feels doomed.

Finally, the patient may be less consciously aware of the event than we would suspect, as Janet (1924) and Breuer and Freud (1925/1955) pointed out more than a half a century ago. Repression and denial are defenses that chase recollection of the noxious event from consciousness and substitute more neutral somatic symptoms. That discovery was the origin of psychoanalysis. Today, the evaluating clinician often infers sexual trauma and/or conflict from projective tests, fantasy material, or the description of the events. However, exploring possible sexual trauma that the child will not reveal is best done by the therapist rather than the evaluator.

Feedback Conferences

The feedback conference with the parents is probably the most difficult part of the evaluation. All the examinations and investigations have been completed. Psychodynamic interpretations are rarely in order at the beginning or even midway in the diagnostic procedure. The clinician has to judge carefully how much psychological explanation can be given at one time without the patient and parents going to another doctor for a more "thorough" medical evaluation.

All members of the team have met and discussed the findings and have come to some tentative hypotheses and recommendations. Now these findings are related to the parents in some palatable way. The family may be more willing to accept that "stress" plays an important role in perpetuating what was initially a "real" physical symptom of an organic disorder. If the child is somatizing and the parents lack insight and are resistant, a simplistic model of stress is often the only feedback that the parents can tolerate. In those families that can see the symptom only in organic terms, collaborative feedback with both the primary care physician and the psychiatrist or psychologist is always best, especially if the parents have trust and confidence in the primary care physician.

In most feedback conferences, some simplified explanation of the mechanisms of conversion or somatization is offered. Perhaps the evaluator correlates the onset of the symptom with some particular stressor. He or she then illustrates how the symptom works out of awareness to resolve the stress, although explaining that this happens outside of conscious volition is difficult. This idea may be easier to integrate than that of secondary gain, which parents often label pejoratively as attention- and sympathy-seeking. The feedback is best given in a positive manner, with confidence that the symptom can be managed. The clinician must often walk a tightrope, explaining the symptom and imparting hope for amelioration through therapy, all without intimating that the patient is manipulative or malingering.

With resistant parents, a specific program that includes physical treatment with the psychotherapy often helps them accept the recommendations. Biofeedback, hypnosis, and physical therapies are more reassuring for the non-psychologically oriented parent than is psychotherapy. Those families who may be willing to participate in psychotherapeutic programs should be given an estimate of the length of time treatment will be required, as well as an idea of the expected outcome. This often makes psychological therapies more acceptable and ultimately more successful.

References

Breuer, J., & Freud, S. (1955). Studies on hysteria. In J. Strachey (Ed. and Trans.). *Standard edition of the complete psychological works of Sigmund Freud* (Vol. 2). London: Hogarth. (Original work published 1925.)

Costello, A.J., Edebrock, C., Kalas, R., Kessler, M.D., & Klarie, S. (1982). *The NIMH diagnostic interview schedule for children, DISC.* Pittsburgh: Author.

Exner, J.E., Jr. (1974). *The Rorschach: A comprehensive system, Vol. 1.* New York: John Wiley & Sons.

Flor-Henry, P., Fromm-Auch, D., Tapper, M., & Schopflocher, D. (1981). A neuropsychological study of the stable syndrome of hysteria. *Biological Psychiatry, 16,* 601–626.

Herjanic, B. (1981). *Psychiatric diagnostic interview for ages 6–17, DSM III version.* St. Louis: Washington University School of Medicine.

Herjanic, B., & Campbell, W. (1977). Differentiating psychiatrically disturbed children on the basis of a structured interview. *Journal of Abnormal Child Psychology, 5,* 127–134.

Janet, P. (1924). *The major symptoms of hysteria*, 2nd Ed., New York: MacMillan.

Kaufman, A.S. (1979). *Intelligent testing with the WISC-R.* New York: John Wiley & Sons.

Puig-Antich, J., & Chambers, W. (1978). *The schedule for affective disorders and schizophrenia for school aged children.* New York: New York State Psychiatric Institute.

Simmons, J. (1983). *Psychiatric examination of children*, 3rd Ed. Philadelphia: Lea and Febiger.

Wasserman, S., & Rosenfeld, A.A (1985). Decision-making in child abuse and neglect. *Bulletin of the American Academy of Psychiatry and Law, 13,* in press.

7

Principles of Clinical Intervention

A variety of therapeutic techniques are available to treat somatoform disorders in children. The appropriate choice depends on: (a) the age of the child, (b) the form and severity of the psychopathology, (c) the psychological milieu of the family, and (d) the type of setting in which the child is being seen. However, in all cases, intervention can be divided into two categories: patient management and specialized treatment techniques (such as biofeedback, hypnosis, medication, and psychotherapy). A practitioner often has difficulty deciding which treatment is most appropriate. Clinicians of widely differing theoretical persuasions promote their own form of intervention as best for all types of somatoform disorders despite the lack of empiric information.

Many therapeutic methods successfully alleviate the symptoms of the disorder. But is that sufficient? Other approaches, such as psychodynamic psychotherapy, have as their goal more fundamental change in the child's personality structure in addition to symptom relief. Despite its apparent desirability, no empiric data exist to support the feasibility or necessity of such a goal for all cases of somatoform disorder.

Outpatient Management

Parents generally deal with symptoms that are normal manifestations of childhood stress (the normal type of transient stress avoider). The cases come to medical attention only when the parents handle the situation very inappropriately, leading to its worsening, or mention it incidentally in a well-child visit. Since primary care physicians, nurse practitioners, school nurses, and parents usually apply general management techniques that prove sufficient to avert further problems, these children rarely see psychologists or psychiatrists.

If during a well-child visit a parent asks how to handle this type of physical symptomatology, the physician may point out that all children occasionally use symptoms to avoid stressful situations. Identifying such symptoms as psychologically induced and making practical suggestions about their handling can also be a great help to inexperienced or insecure parents. For example, parents of children with vague recurrent symptoms such as stomachache or headache can be counseled to set clear-cut rules about when their child is allowed to stay home. Pediatricians are well aware that vomiting, anorexia, fever, or diarrhea almost always accompany serious abdominal pathology. Similarly, the child who complains of a headache accompanied by vomiting, visual changes, stiff neck, photophobia, or fever must be treated quite differently from the child who, after hopping out of bed and eating breakfast, announces that he or she has a headache and does not want to go to school, while running over to watch TV. Thus, the parent can be taught to help differentiate organic pain from a functional disturbance by learning to pay attention to accompanying behavior or symptoms. Parents also should be counseled to acknowledge minor physical injuries and to comfort their child without dwelling on the injury or becoming overly solicitous. Ideally, parents should discuss physical complaints in a manner appropriate to the true severity of the illness. Unfortunately, some parents become infantile and histrionic. It is important to remember that different cultural subgroups have different ideas about what is appropriate when confronting their child's minor illness. In general, warmth and nurturance help a child who is hurt; exaggerating the symptomatology may actually frighten the child.

In some pediatric cases, the organic symptom becomes the parent's "conversion symptom." The parent (most frequently, but not exclusively, the mother) who tends to focus on the child's mild symptomatology and makes multiple calls to the physician about medically insignificant problems may be anxious about an unrelated issue. If she is unable to express her feelings, the anxiety may be translated instead into a focus on the child's physical symptoms. In one case, no amount of reassurance would convince the mother that her newborn infant's mild colicky symptoms would disappear by themselves within the next few weeks. After many urgent phone calls and several unnecessary visits, the mother confided that her husband had not wanted a baby and was theatening to leave her. In other cases, the symptom is the parent's way of gaining access to professional attention. One mother made repeated visits to her pediatrician, unsatisfied that her daughter's viral illness was properly diagnosed. After several visits, she broke down in tears and told her pediatrician that her real concern was about serious marital difficulties. In this situation, the parent uses the child's mild organic pain or illness as a vehicle to discharge her own anxiety.

Some parents lack the personal resources or support system that would enable them to contain, ease, or discharge their anxiety. In such cases, confiding to the pediatrician is beneficial; it breaks the focus on the child whose minor organic symptom will be allowed to disappear naturally with no sequelae. The anxiety is properly focused, and steps can be taken to deal with it. These cases are clearly related to the stress level of the parent and are not reflective of the child's anxiety. If the parent is handled with sensitivity and appropriate crisis management, the pattern of somatization will have been avoided.

In other cases where this pattern is more entrenched, the parent is unable to express his or her own anxiety directly, and the focus on the child's somatic symptom results from the parent's inability to express affect directly. Cases of the first type require sensitivity and crisis management for the parent. For those of the second type, specific management techniques are required.

If this vicious cycle of minor childhood ailments leading to major medical attention continues, the child grows up unable to discriminate between serious and minor complaints. And it is precisely in these families that are unable to deal with psychological problems in any way other than through physical attention in which the child learns that saying that something hurts is the only way to get attention when a problem of any type arises.

When a child presents with mild somatoform complaints, an alert clinician who is aware of the differential diagnosis can plan effective interventions that will prevent milder symptoms from becoming entrenched and elaborated. The primary care physician can take charge of and effectively deal with mild somatoform syndromes such as mild polysymptomatic disorder (Type 1, described in Chapter 5). This is particularly true when secondary gain appears to be the prime motivation, when the stressors present are neither severe, traumatic, nor irreversible, when the child is relatively young, and when no previous psychiatric history exists.

However, more serious symptoms often have many determinants and serve defensive functions that are crucial to the child's and the family's homeostasis. No simple interventions will rid the patient of them. These more serious and persistent symptoms should be referred to a skilled clinician experienced in working with children and families.

Several general guidelines may help the primary care physician and other clinicians to properly manage somatoform disorders.

1. *Consider psychological factors early and minimize medical procedures.* When children who have no obvious psychopathology show up in the pediatrician's or general practitioner's office with recurrent headaches, stomachaches, or neurologic symptoms, the physician must consider at the outset the possibility that these symptoms are the result of psychological stress. Obviously, if the history and findings on physical examination could be compatible with a particular disease process, those medical tests that are required to rule out disease must be performed. However, as the old saying goes, "When you hear hoofbeats, think of horses, not zebras!" If psychological factors are suspected, the physician must be careful not to suggest an excessive medical workup. For instance, if all clues point to somatoform disorder as the cause of a child's headache, cerebral angiography to rule out transient ischemic attacks is unnecessary and unwise. Such a workup can be dangerous, expensive, and painful. In addition, an increasing number of medical procedures to rule out more and more esoteric diagnoses diverts the patient and his or her family away from obvious psychological factors and reinforces their tendency to somatize to cope with or avoid dealing with stress.

Many physicians do not prepare the family until after an excessive and exhaustive search for organic factors has turned out negative. In these cases, if the physician says, "I can't find anything wrong. It must be psychologically based," the family will feel that this doctor must have missed something since he or she was convinced enough of an organic etiology to do all those tests. Maybe another doctor won't miss the answer, and the family often begins all over again with another primary physician, rather than finally seeking the psychological assistance they need.

Alternatively, if the physician explains early in the diagnostic process that psychological factors frequently produce or exacerbate symptomatology, the family will be forewarned of the possibility that factors that are not purely organic may ultimately play some role in explaining this condition. They will not later feel that the doctor has simply settled for the diagnosis because of failure to find the real organic cause. Once the necessary medical tests are completed and the findings are negative, the physician needs to be definitive about physical problems being absent, explaining to the parents that although the symptoms are real and painful, they have a psychological origin. This concept is often difficult for laypersons to accept, and the explanation should be given in a way that does not minimize the symptom or demean the parents' concern about it. They must be told that psychological symptoms are real, not imaginary, and may be associated with both psychological and physical pain. The pain is the same; the method of treatment differs.

During patient visits, the physician ought to turn the conversation to factors in the child's life other than the somatic complaints. This is a deliberate strategy to shift the focus towards stress and psychological factors. For example, by asking questions about school performance and social relationships, the physician is trying to help parents understand that these factors are important in their child's development. Asking parents to describe the child's psychological development and characteristics may help the physician get a better perspective on how psychologically-minded the parents are while helping them focus on becoming more educated about these issues. If the physician senses strong resistance to a psychological explanation, it might help to suggest that a diagnostic opinion regarding the role of psychological factors might help clarify the situation. Since some parents and children need time and gentle suggestion before they can accept the possibility of a psychological etiology for the symptoms, immediate referral for psychotherapy will often scare the parents off. Recommending a psychiatric and/or psychological diagnostic consultation as part of the evaluative process will more often lead to cooperation. The more tentative approach is preferred and is more often successful.

2. *Minimize secondary gain*. The physician needs to explain carefully and nonjudgmentally that the child ultimately benefits if the parents focus on what the child is capable of and not on what the child cannot do. Specifically, the physician must give parents guidelines so that they reinforce the child's participation in social and school activities, ignore talking about physical symptoms, and ask few questions about physical symptomatology, thereby minimizing the secondary gain the child might be getting from other family members and peers. As part of this education, parents must be helped to understand the significance of various symptoms. It is helpful for the physician to describe the type of physical symptoms for which he or she wishes to be called, as well as those that can safely be discussed at the next scheduled appointment, not before.

However, even children with psychogenic symptoms, such as the headaches and stomachaches typical of school avoidance behavior, can develop appendicitis or meningitis. Parents must be carefully instructed to call their physician if the symptom or its severity changes or if they suspect that something different is going on.

If the symptoms interfere with schooling, the physician must encourage the parents to send the child back to school unless a legitimate reason precludes it. If the parents cannot set limits, the physician must develop rules for when the child can legitimately miss school, preferably in collaboration with the school nurse (or whoever makes decisions about excuses from class or school). Physicians and nurses must delineate and enforce the guidelines that the child, school, and parents must follow. For example, if the child comes to school and complains of headache, the nurse (a) may administer an acetominophen, (b) may let the child lie down for up to half an hour, and then (c) must send the child back to class. Work that is missed must be made up entirely.

3. *Identify and reduce environmental stress*. In mild cases, a particular stress is often difficult to pinpoint. Some of the common causes of childhood stress include general problems involving specific developmental crises. These include schoolage issues such as performance difficulties and frustration with schoolwork, transitions to junior or senior high school, and pubertal issues around sexual development. Such difficulties are especially common among children with concomitant learning disorders. The child's stress may also stem from a family problem, parental marital difficulty, a death, a move, or some other separation crisis. Once the stress is identified, simple interventions should be undertaken if possible. The clinician must then decide whether changes that involve parent or teacher guidance, reassurance, and changes in school environment are sufficient to ameliorate the situation or whether a referral should be made to a psychiatrist or psychologist. Since referral may be costly and can make parents feel inadequate, it is not entirely benign. If the referral undermines their confidence in their ability to parent, the child may well suffer. Therefore, referrals should be considered judiciously, but made unambiguously when clearly indicated.

At some point, preferably early in the evaluative process, it is important for the physician to talk to the child alone to inquire about the child's understanding of his or her symptoms and their causes. Sometimes it is easy to identify the stress by finding out what was happening or was about to happen when the symptoms began.

We have seen one 9-year-old extremely bright obese boy who has had years of stomach pains unaccompanied by anorexia, fever, vomiting, diarrhea, or constipation. He was under obvious tremendous pressure to perform from parents who were superachievers. Despite his IQ of 155, he was being tutored for his "learning disabilities." When asked what was the thing he was most afraid of that might be the cause of his recurrent pain, he answered, "Not enough homework." This child's pains of long-standing duration disappeared shortly after beginning family psychotherapy.

4. *Direct symptom control*. Once the stressful situation is identified, the child must be helped to find some other ways of coping with the stress. For example,

the child can be helped to develop some verbal self-monitoring—things the child can say to himself or herself to ease the stress. In *The King and I*, Anna, teaching her pupils to sing "Whenever I feel afraid, I whistle a happy tune," provides a perfect example of this type of approach. Sometimes during the process if the school nurse explores the stressor (test, teasing, reprimand, worry about home, etc.) with the child, the child can then be sent back to the class without even being given the analgesic, which is preferable since the child begins to realize, however dimly, that talking can make some painful symptoms go away without pharmacologic intervention. The combination of understanding and firmness is often difficult to implement, particularly in a situation where the physician's insight into a symptom's function is hazy. However, the parents of a child who regularly uses somatization to cope should not be called to take the child home unless the symptomatology is significant or the pattern is atypical for this child.

At times, the symptom serves a function that is so important psychologically that the patient resists efforts to treat and eliminate it. The therapist is often caught between wanting to help the child to quickly be rid of a debilitating symptom and understanding that care must be taken because the child needs the symptom for emotional protection. Since removing the precipitating conflict can be a long tedious process, many authorities recommend that the clinician try to alleviate the symptom when he or she has determined that no serious psychological risk is involved in removing the defense. In Type 1 cases, it is important not to overtreat, but to deal with the presenting physical symptomatology in a matter-of-fact way to make the patient feel that the clinician is attending to it and recognizes it as legitimate. Judicious use of analgesics, muscle relaxants, compresses, and other simple remedies along with direct suggestion may well suffice. In some cases, referral for some form of psychological treatment such as relaxation therapy or biofeedback may be appropriate. These treatments will be discussed in the next section.

Patients who are not motivated for psychotherapy, who are not severely stressed, or who have a limited capacity for insight do not usually benefit from psychodynamically oriented psychotherapy. Short-term, reality-oriented, directive counseling may be effective in educating the child and helping him or her find some alternative strategies for coping. However, parents who lack psychological-mindedness and reinforce the somatization may make it difficult to help the child change. In these cases, a necessary adjunct to the child's counseling is supportive guidance for the parents.

Management on a Pediatric Ward

Children with Type 2 disorders (monosymptomatic somatization disorders) often undergo multiple complex inpatient medical workups. Needless to say, many of these children present particularly difficult management problems. Since somatoform symptoms often start with an actual physical illness whose symptoms persist long after they should have disappeared, the child and the family are asked to make subtle distinctions between the initial organic illness that caused the symptom and its evolution into a symptom maintained by psychological factors. Symptoms that at first were signs of a physical illness, such as the flu or infectious mononucleosis, have lingered and transmuted because they became important vehicles for alleviating the child's and often the family's emotional stress. Even the physician may find it difficult to sort out the lingering effects of a physical illness from the manifestations of psychological distress.

These children's parents often believe deeply that a physical disease continues to afflict their child. Therefore, they resist any psychological explanation, even one introduced as a possibility at the very beginning of the diagnostic process. If management is not done in a fashion that is sensitive to the family's needs and beliefs, the parents will sometimes continue to doctor-shop. Confrontation rarely works; it leads many patients to feel that the health care professionals doubt their veracity or consider them ignorant and inferior. Physicians cannot simply make psychological symptoms disappear by explaining them rationally: a clinician is well advised never to tell a patient that his or her symptoms are not real nor to imply that the symptoms are imaginary or "all in the patient's head." The child who hears this often begins to worry that the doctor thinks he or she is crazy. This is disrespectful and will often break whatever therapeutic alliance has developed.

To respect a patient also means respecting the fact the patient has symptoms for a reason. To say to a patient, "Don't have your symptoms because they're all in your head," is to say, "I don't respect that your psychological processes have a meaning, especially if you are unaware of that meaning." Although letting the child keep some of the physical symptomatology and employing some physical methods of treating the symptoms may at times seem like hocus-pocus, it can be a critical factor that ensures a continuing alliance with the patient and the family. Over time, that alliance may allow the clinician to deal with the psychological issues.

These hospitalized children and their parents often have personality disorders. Dependent and histrionic personality patterns are frequent. Thus, secondary gain motivates much of the dependent child's behavior; somatization is the ticket to nurturance in the family. "Doctoring" is a life style for many of these families. For the histrionic child, giving up the symptoms means sacrificing the attention the child needs and the gratification he or she can get in no other way. This behavior pattern often works against the successful treatment of these disorders.

The pediatric neurologist, the pediatric house staff, the pediatric psychologist, and the child psychiatrist are the professionals most likely to evaluate and treat such patients. Some guidelines for intervening with a patient undergoing an extensive inpatient workup are as follows.

The first priority is to investigate the possibility that the etiology is organic. That goal should be reached as quickly and efficiently as possible. Psychiatric and/or psychological evaluation should be a part of every workup and should be done at the outset. These patients and their families need to realize from the beginning that psychological factors are being considered. Since this strategy also prepares the house staff and legitimizes psychologically caused illnesses, it can frequently prevent their feeling angry that the patient is malingering or in some way fooling them if the workup yields no clear cut organic etiology.

Secondary gain is often difficult to minimize in the hospital. As a rule, hospital staff focuses on somatic symptoms and often resist requiring patients to be involved in caring for themselves. If these patients are to begin to improve, they must not be allowed to stay in bed or avoid ward activities such as recreation, school, or other programs. Parents need to be counseled to spend much of their time with the child, focusing their conversation on subjects other than symptoms. Specific orders need to be written that encourage normal activities. If the patient is discharged after a thorough medical workup proves negative, rehospitalization is recommended only if new developments make it essential.

Points of stress should be identified with the help of a psychological or psychiatric consultant who sometimes also provides the appropriate intervention. This clinician needs regular contact with the patient to develop a relationship that will allow the patient to share his or her fears, worries, and problems. Beginning psychotherapy while the patient is an inpatient will often secure a relationship and allow the patient to reveal traumatic events in a safe environment. Sometimes, if time is short, hypnosis and relaxation techniques can be helpful (Spiegel & Rosenfeld, 1984). In the older literature many practitioners endorsed the use of sodium amytal interviews as a way of helping patients relax their defenses and reveal traumatic precipitants if they exist (Forbis & Jones, 1965; Proctor, 1958; Stevens, 1969), but this technique is not currently in great favor because of its physical and psychological invasiveness.

Long-term psychological treatment is strongly recommended. The revelation of the trauma, if one existed, is rarely sufficient since the conflict still exists and the child needs to incorporate new ways of dealing with the feelings that the event generated. Psychotherapy for such patients is described briefly in the next section.

The hospital is often a good place to begin treatment to alleviate the presenting symptom. The following are some widely accepted methods for symptom relief for children with somatoform symptoms.

Direct Suggestion

A specific plan should be presented to the patient and the family. It should include a description of the psychological and medical treatments that are planned, specific recommendations for activities, such as return to school complete with a timetable for both part-time and full-time return. In some cases, the activity being avoided is one the child abhors. The need for the activity should be reevaluated. For instance, one sensitive boy had to be hospitalized because he suffered severe bilateral leg weakness. In the course of an extensive workup, he intimated that he did not want to play football, a game his athletic father was pushing vigorously. In this case, the boy needed an ally since he could not say no overtly. When his physician told both the boy and his parents that his condition, although serious, would slowly improve, but that contact sports would have to be avoided for the foreseeable future, the boy began improving and ultimately regained full use of his legs. In this way, the boy's need to avoid these sports was respected, while giving both he and his father the acceptable out that this boy sadly was too ill to play them.

Setting concrete dates for accomplishing specific goals often serves as a direct suggestion to the patient. Although occasionally, a child is ready for full-time return to school immediately, a more gradual introduction diminishes the possibility that the plan will fail suddenly and that the symptom will recur. A specific course for the symptoms should be suggested; for example, partial relief by discharge and full relief within a specified period of time, perhaps by the time the patient comes for a follow-up visit. Concrete suggestions should be made to parents about their involvement and help.

Physical Therapies

Physical symptoms, especially those that debilitate the patient, often must be dealt with. Physical therapy for paralysis, weakness, and pain is often helpful, particularly if the physical therapist is familiar with somatizing patients and discourages secondary gain. When a physical illness has preceded the somatization problem, this is especially helpful. Physical therapy, when prescribed, should be one component of a larger package of recommendations that includes psychological treatment.

Medication

We could find no references in the literature about using psychotropic medication to treat somatoform disorders, nor have we found these medications useful as a regular treatment. Psychological symptoms that accompany these disorders, such as depression and anxiety, might be treated with antidepressants or antianxiety medications. However, because these patients are so strongly focused on the organic factors that might be causing their symptoms, psychological treatment is more likely than psychotropic medication to help the patient come to grips with the psychological stresses that he or she is avoiding.

On occasion, we use analgesics and muscle relaxants rather than psychotropic medications to accompany psychological treatment, especially in cases where the patient has a large investment in them, a deep belief in their efficacy, and has agreed to a plan for decreasing their use.

Relaxation Therapy

Relaxation treatments often help children who suffer both pain and weakness. Relaxation training has been used in conjunction with biofeedback, hypnosis, or psychotherapy, or as a treatment modality in and of itself. Originating in the 1930s, progressive relaxation training was developed by Jacobson (1938), who used alternate tensing and releasing of specific muscles to help the patient with chronic anxiety learn to deeply relax. Wolpe (1958) modified Jacobson's techniques for use in his systematic desensitization procedures, which employed relaxation as an incompatible response with anxiety. Bernstein and Borkovec (1973) developed a widely used systematic progressive relaxation method. Their manual for progressive relaxation training marked a systematic presentation of the technique with applications for specific symptoms such as insomnia, for somatic illnesses caused by tension, and for enhancing psychotherapy. Their techniques involves a series of steps: (a) focusing attention on the muscle, (b) tensing the muscle, (c) maintaining tension for 5 to 7 seconds, (d) releasing tension, and (e) maintaining attention on the relaxing muscle. This sequence is done with 16 muscle groups. The patient is encouraged to practice twice a day.

In conjunction with physical therapy, biofeedback, and psychotherapies, progressive relaxation therapy often helps children with conversion and somatization disorders. It is easily taught in the hospital environment, where frequent supervised practice sessions are possible. Patients are helped to develop increased attention to and discrimination between body sensations. The technique is also a process over which the patient has control (especially control independent of parent involvement). Some therapists have found relaxation exercises useful during interviews to decrease defensiveness and anxiety, thus encouraging self-disclosure.

However, relaxation techniques seem to be less useful as the sole intervention technique. Anxiety is a signal; psychological defenses exist because they serve an important psychological function. Attenuating the debilitation they cause can be helpful, but the price is often unknown. Therefore, relaxation is recommended as an adjunct but not as replacement for psychotherapy.

Hypnosis

Hypnotic techniques have long been used with adult patients with somatoform disorders. Because the hypnotized patient is in a hypersuggestible state when the trance is induced, posthypnotic suggestion sometimes can be employed to rid the patient of the symptom. Hypnosis can also be a useful tool for exploring possible traumatic precipitants of the symptom, allowing the events that led to the conversion symptom developing to be clarified.

In these cases, hypnosis is not entirely safe. Possible dangers include symptom substitution, encouragement of dependency, exploitation of the patient because of their heightened suggestibility, and severe anxiety as a reaction to both the process and the insights gained. Guarding the patient from these dangers requires a great deal of experience and training. Hypnosis and hypnotherapy are techniques that require expertise and training that are beyond the scope of this book to provide (see Spiegel & Spiegel, 1978).

Biofeedback

Biofeedback has been used primarily to alleviate headache and pain. Its use in the treatment of headache, the history of its development, and a review of current literature are covered in Chapter 8. However, no references could be found using biofeedback for other conversion and somatization symptoms. Mostofsky and Balaschak (1977) discussed the use of biofeedback with epileptic patients; the treatment has some application to pseudoseizures. However, no specific studies of such patients have been done. Although our experience is limited to a handful of cases, we have found biofeedback in combination with psychotherapy to be an aid in alleviating children's somatoform symptoms.

Biofeedback is self-regulation via auditory or visual feedback of a body condition such as temperature or muscle tension. Through visualization, imagery, and self-suggestion, patients learn to warm their hands; through relaxation and self-suggestion, they learn to reduce muscle contraction, thus reducing electrical conduction across the muscle as measured by electromyogram (EMG). Biofeedback by EMG can be of help to patients with specific contraction, pain, or paralysis in a localized region of the body.

Biofeedback has several major advantages in children with somatoform symptoms: (a) It is perceived as more organic or more physical; thus, patients who resist psychological explanations respond more positively to it. (b) It is structured and concrete, and the expectation for the patient's behavior is simple and understandable. The patient is not expected to do anything very complex or vague. (c) The visual feedback recommended for these cases may be more concrete and helpful since these patients may have some difficulty with complex and subtle linguistic input. (d) These patients may be quite suggestible and, thus, will be compliant and improve because they are supposed to. The placebo effect is quite strong medicine whose primary side effect is the projection of some magical powers onto the clinician. (e) We hypothesized in Chapter 3 that these patients may, as a baseline, have poor somatosensory discrimination, may inhibit perception of sensory afferent stimuli, or may be inattentive to sensory afferents. Biofeedback is a technique that teaches the patient either to attend to or to discriminate between sensory stimuli. (f) These patients are remarkably ignorant of the possibilities of cognitive control over their body functions. Biofeedback can help patients learn that they control such functions, rather than depend on control coming from external sources. (g) Biofeedback can also be used as a structured way to begin a therapeutic alliance. Once the symptom is gone, if the therapist has been involved regularly with the biofeedback (even if only in monitoring it), the transition to psychotherapy may be easier since the patient is pleased that the therapist has proven that he or she can do something concrete to help. In addition, relaxation techniques, which are often part of the biofeedback training, also facilitate the patient's relaxation of defenses and can provide another transition to psychotherapy.

The following is a case report of treatment at the University of Minnesota, Division of Pediatric Neurology, using a combined biofeedback and a short-term psychotherapy approach. The history and diagnostic considerations for this case can be found in Chapter 5.

Lane is a 16-year-old boy with a conversion dysphagia (inability to swallow). His mother overprotects him; this overprotection has contributed to Lane's feeling angry at and helpless in the world. He did not feel in control of his life. At least by not eating, he could control one area. He was seen for 1 hour per week for combined therapy, involving EMG biofeedback to reduce throat tension and short-term psychotherapy to focus on self-reliance issues.

The first biofeedback session was used to acclimate Lane to the equipment and demonstrate through the use of a visual monitor how tension adversely affected his ability to swallow. He was provided with an elementary explanation of how the three electrodes placed around his throat would pick up electrical impulses in the surrounding muscles and register them on the CRT screen. By the end of the first session, he was quite successful in controlling the tension. The succeeding sessions consisted of an initial relaxation period, followed by Lane eating a specific type of food chosen for its consistency and texture. Foods were chosen to provide gradually increasing firmness. When the tension in his throat increased, Lane would practice relaxing his throat to facilitate swallowing. He was also given a homework assignment each week to try one type of food that he had previously been unable to eat. By the end of the seventh session, Lane was able to eat all foods, although somewhat slowly. After biofeedback therapy ended on the seventh week, the entire hour was devoted to psychotherapy.

Lane appeared to be a depressed, passive-dependent adolescent. His father was emotionally distant, and his mother supplied nurturance for his medical but not for his emotional discomforts. As a result of his swallowing difficulties, Lane's dependence on his family increased and resulted in his receiving additional attention from family members (secondary gain).

Psychotherapy focused on promoting Lane's self-reliance and reinforcing his perception, albeit limited, that some things in the environment were within his control, such as swallowing. Problem-solving exercises centered around current life stresses were conducted as a means of teaching Lane strategies for dealing with day to day problems along with encouraging a sense of mastery. Appropriate ways to express anger (as opposed to internalizing it) were also explored. Unfortunately, insurance coverage allowed only 10 sessions. Given the limited time constraints, no attempt was made to deal directly with the issues that underlay his depression.

Lane's perception of his problem changed during the course of treatment. He initially stated that his trouble with swallowing was something he had to learn to live with. At the end of treatment, Lane stated that his problem with swallowing was related to tension, and that from prior experiences in the biofeedback lab, he knew he could now control it. At the end of therapy, Lane was eating normal foods at home and was less isolated socially.

Psychotherapy

Since psychological trauma, not physical illness, is more likely to precede conversion reaction cases in which specific symptoms have a symbolic meaning to the patient, the clinician's job is somewhat easier. The physical symptoms in these cases often do not conform to what is anatomically possible, nor is a history of multiple physical symptomatology seen. Frequently, some crisis (often sexual abuse) can be identified either in the family or in the patient.

When the symptom is the response to serious trauma, persistent, thoughtful, and uncritical inquiries may help the child talk about the experience and keep the emotions he or she has connected to it from being bottled-up inside. Repeated visits are often necessary for trust to develop and for the child to be able to talk about the trauma, but the child must make this decision to talk or show in play what happened. If the clinician is aggressive in pushing the child to talk, it can feel to the child like another intrusive attack similar to the initial trauma. Patience is, therefore, paramount. The child may benefit from a psychological or psychiatric consultation aimed at discovering the best way to help the child deal with the traumatic event and integrate it emotionally. Such work takes time, but may very well help prevent further symptoms from developing now or later. When either physical or sexual abuse has caused the symptom, the child may be afraid or embarrassed. The physician must decide whether such a trauma might have occurred. If the clinician strongly suspects that it has, reporting is mandatory and referral warranted. Guidelines for evaluating and managing molested children are available elsewhere (Rosenfeld, 1979).

Since parents in conversion cases are usually less resistant to the psychological explanation of symptoms, they are more likely to follow referral recommendations. However, the parents may have a hard time handling the disorder's physical manifestations, which may be severe enough to prevent the patient from functioning. The parents need to know the psychological stress can cause physical symptoms that are real, not imaginary, and that require psychological treatment to heal them.

Some experts recommend a two-step procedure for treating such cases, which entails, first, removing the symptoms, and second, individual psychotherapy. Others feel that a single psychological intervention is preferable and that symptoms are best removed solely through the psychotherapeutic process.

In the two-step procedure, a variety of methods aid the therapist in removing the symptom, including direct suggestion, relaxation and hypnosis, and biofeedback. After or simultaneous with symptom removal, psychotherapy is initiated, paying specific attention to the emotional aspects of the precipitating stressor or traumatic event.

Psychotherapy using a psychoanalytic or psychodynamic model is particularly appropriate for the older child with a conversion disorder when the symptom is a neurotic one. For younger children, the goal and healing force is not necessarily insight. Nevertheless, the therapist is most effective if he or she keeps in mind the underlying psychodynamic factors producing the symptoms.

Conversion symptoms arise out of conflict. They represent the individual's attempt to deal with the discomfort that comes from the presence of unacceptable feelings or wishes. However, developing a symptom does not always fully resolve the conflict; the symptom often makes the child feel weak or helpless, and the attempt to bind anxiety with the symptom is often insufficient or exacts too high a price in diminished functioning. Secondary gain, even though present, is not very compelling for these children since the trauma they have experienced overwhelms them and compromises a personality that has functioned well in the past. In these cases, the child is strongly motivated to resolve the conflict and reduce the anxiety.

For these patients with conversion reactions, the goal of psychotherapy is to make the conflict conscious. When the patient becomes aware of the feelings underlying the symptom, he or she can explore them and can often master the conflict without sacrificing function. Understanding the emotions that cause the symptoms and being able to bear them help the patient create more effective problem-solving strategies while increasing the patient's sense of mastery and self-esteem.

Specific psychotherapeutic techniques are too numerous and complex to address here. There are a few things to consider when embarking on insight-oriented psychotherapy with these children. Great difficulty starting in therapy and producing any material in the therapeutic hour are a frequent problem. The patient may focus on somatic symptoms rather than on psychological issues, and dependency needs often intrude. Resistance to insight may be very strong because the child is unaware of the nature of the conflict. The patient may actively resist the therapist's interpretations at first, even if he or she is aware of what is conflictual.

Many children with conversion reactions have an inordinate need to be "good." This wish affects therapy because the child resists revealing any feelings, fantasies, or thoughts that he or she fears can be construed as "bad." Sexual urges and experiences, when seen as manifestations of the patient's badness, give rise to pervasive guilt. Sexual impulses and desires may be denied entirely or projected onto others. To the patient, being "good" may also mean not expressing angry feelings; for some girls, it may mean excessively feminine behavior or it can mean not having any feelings. Because these children seek approval constantly, they often ask the therapist, "What do you want me to do?" One helpful answer is, "To be yourself." The message is, "I want you to be all that you are, not to be just the parts you think I would approve of."

One of the most common problems in psychotherapy of children with conversion reactions is that inexperienced therapists too rapidly interpret the child's defenses and conflicts. Although the child's words and self-awareness make rapid interpretation tempting, as we said earlier, this overlooks the fact that defenses are there for a reason and that too early exposure may be experienced by the child as an intrusion on his or her privacy. Not surprisingly, the patient often flees from interpretations that seem obvious to the therapist. Patience is necessary in treating these cases. Over time, a gradual desensitization takes place through an incorporation of the therapist's attitude that "good" and "bad" are not the central issue. The patient comes to terms with who he or she is and, in abuse cases, with disturbing experiences that may have been overwhelming and confusing. With treatment, debilitating defenses and undeserved guilt subside in many cases, and more mature strategies that involve more rational and thoughtful ways of coping with impulses emerge. Rather than feeling controlled by unseen forces, the individual is less easily overwhelmed and controls himself or herself to a far greater extent. Self-esteem grows as the child gains the conviction that he or she now has the inner strength to master conflicts that will arise in the future.

Obviously, psychotherapy requires special skills. With younger children, experience in doing play therapy (conversing through cars and dolls) is essential. With less intelligent, less introspective adolescents whose goals and capacity for insight are often more limited, psychotherapy is more difficult. In addition to helping the child accept his or her feelings, the therapist must help the child develop alternative coping strategies to repression and somatization, occasionally suggesting alternative concrete ways to deal with the feelings and anxieties specific situations elicit. When circumstances militate against long-term psychotherapy, these more limited goals can often be achieved.

Psychiatric Hospitalization and Other More Intensive Treatment

For the patient with severe somatization disorder, secondary gain is more important than primary gain in maintaining the symptoms. The pathology is pervasive in and belongs to the entire family in which somatic symptoms are the norm. Thus, outpatient insight-oriented psychotherapy rarely works in these cases because both the child and the family system are so resistant and problematic. Sometimes placement in a therapeutic milieu is the only way to treat such cases successfully.

Without early and intensive intervention, children with somatization disorder are thought to be at risk for developing Briquet's syndrome or debilitating lifelong physical complaints (Ernst, Routh, & Harper, 1984; Robins & O'Neal, 1953). Since these children are frequently admitted to hospitals, psychiatric consultation should be obtained early and speedy transfer to a psychiatric facility made when indicated. Because the symptoms are so severe, psychiatric hospitalization or residential treatment may be the only effective method of intervention. Family influences, whether genetic or environmental, seem to play a strong role in these cases. The families have multiple problems; the men are often violent and alcoholic, and the women have histories of multiple somatic complaints and personality disorders (Bohman, Cloninger, von Knorring, & Sigvardsson, 1984; Cloninger, Reich, & Guze, 1975; Spalt, 1980). Although we have rarely seen such polysymptomatic patients before adolescence, when we have, treatment was difficult because the secondary gain was such a compelling factor and the accompanying personality disorders were so pervasive. Although we have recommended intensive inpatient programs with a strong milieu in such cases, outcomes are uncertain, even when intervention is made early.

References

Bernstein, D.A., & Borkovec, T.D. (1973). *Progressive relaxation training*. Champaign, IL: Research Press.

Bohman, M., Cloninger, R., von Knorring, A., & Sigvardsson, S. (1984). An adoption study of somatoform disorders: III. Cross-fostering analysis and genetic relationships to alcoholism and criminality. *Archives of General Psychiatry, 41*, 872–878.

Cloninger, C.R., Reich, T., & Guze, S. (1975). The multifactorial model of disease transmission: III. Familial relationship between sociopathy and hysteria (Briquet's syndrome). *British Journal of Psychiatry, 127*, 23–32.

Ernst, A.R., Routh, D.K., & Harper, D. (1984). Abdominal pain in children and symptoms of somatization disorder. *Journal of Pediatric Psychology, 9*, 77–86.

Forbis, O.L., & Jones, R.H. (1965). Hysteria in childhood. *Southern Medical Journal, 58*, 1221.

Jacobsen, E. (1938). *Progressive relaxation*. Chicago: University of Chicago Press.

Moss, C.S. (1965). *Hypnosis in perspective*. New York: Macmillan.

Mostofsky, D., & Balaschak, B.A. (1977). Psychobiological control of seizures. *Psychological Bulletin, 84*, 723–750.

Proctor, J.T. (1958). Hysteria in childhood. *American Journal of Orthopsychiatry, 28*, 394–407.

Robins, E., & O'Neal, P. (1953). Clinical features of hysteria in children—with a note on prognosis: A two to seventeen year follow-up study of 41 patients. *Nervous Child, 10*, 246–271.

Rosenfeld, A.A (1979). The clinical management of incest and sexual abuse of children. *Journal of the American Medical Association, 242*, 1761–1764.

Spalt, L. (1980). Hysteria and antisocial personality. *Journal of Nervous and Mental Disease, 168*, 456–464.

Spiegel, D., & Rosenfeld, A.A (1984). Spontaneous hypnotic age regression: Case report. *Journal of Clinical Psychiatry, 45*, 522–524.

Spiegel, H., & Spiegel, D. (1978). *Trance and treatment. Clinical uses of hypnosis*. New York: Basic Books.

Stevens, H. (1969). Conversion hysteria—revisited by the pediatric neurologist. *Clinical Proceedings of Childrens Hospital of Washington DC, 25*, 27–39.

Wolpe, J. (1958). *Psychotherapy by reciprocal inhibition*. Stanford: Stanford University Press.

8

Headache in Children: Diagnosis and Treatment

While the distinction between conversion and psychogenic pain disorder in DSM III may be useful in adults, because of the frequent coexistence of pain with other nonpain symptoms in children, it is quite arbitrary. Psychogenic pain symptoms in children are primarily abdominal pain or headache. Several authors have noted that abdominal pain is more frequently seen in younger children and headache more frequent in older children (Oster, 1972). It appears that some children with somatization disorder progress from abdominal pain to headache as they grow older. A rather extensive literature is available on psychogenic abdominal pain in children (Apley, 1975; Christensen & Mortenson, 1975; Farrell, 1984; Stone & Barbero, 1970). There is also substantial literature on headache. Because headache is a frequent symptom in somatization disorders, occurs as a conversion symptom, is the most common somatoform symptom across all age groups, and the differential diagnosis includes other psychologically important diagnosis such as migraine, tension headache, and depression, we will address it more fully here.

Despite the high frequency with which headache is a chief complaint to the primary care physician, its diagnosis and treatment in children remain a relatively neglected subject. Many times, children's headaches are simply treated with bed rest or over-the-counter analgesics such as aspirin and acetaminophen. However, recent investigations have demonstrated that all forms of headache occur in prepubertal children and that many require more specialized forms of treatment similar to those available to adults.

This chapter reviews recent literature on the assessment and treatment of headaches. We define the types of headaches that occur in children, address issues of differential diagnosis, discuss the epidemiology of various headache types, and give the long-term prognosis for juvenile-onset headache. Although various treatment approaches are discussed, we will focus on the development of biofeedback techniques to relieve headache pain, and describe typical biofeedback procedures in a case example that demonstrates how these procedures can be used with a child.

This chapter was written by Norman Cohen.

While neither migraine nor tension headache are usually classified as a somatoform disorder, we will include both in this chapter since they are the two most studied and most common types of headaches and often overlap with somatoform headaches. Although they may be precipitated or exacerbated by psychological factors, physiologic change contributes in whole or in part to the etiology of either type of headache. In the case of migraine, this involves vascular processes; for tension headaches, this involves head or neck muscle contraction for relatively prolonged periods (e.g., several hours, days, or weeks). Often, however, psychogenic or conversion headache coexists with migraine or is hard to distinguish from tension headache. Headache, as a conversion symptom or as a symptom of a somatization disorder, shares many characteristics with and is often difficult to distinguish from migraine and tension headaches. Thus, the criteria, incidence, causative factors, and treatment of various headache syndromes may overlap.

Definitions of Headache

Two distinct types of headache have been known for many centuries. Tension headache (also called muscle contraction headache, common headache) is undoubtedly the most common type. Despite its almost universal prevalence, no precise definition is available. In contrast, migraines have been distinguishable from common headaches since the ancient Greeks, who defined migraine headache as a particularly severe headache with sudden onset, usually focused on one side of the head, and often accompanied by visual phenomenon occurring before the sharp pain. Bille (1962) cited a 200-year old classification of headaches into "common headache" and migraines, "a disease entity different from common headaches" (p. 22).

Recently a number of investigators have attempted more specific definitions of migraine. The first to attempt a brief definition derived from observed symptoms was Vahlquist (1955). He postulated that all migraines involved recurrent paroxysmal headaches with extended asymptomatic intervals between attacks. He further stated that to be diagnosed as having migraines, an individual would have to have two of four other symptoms: nausea and/or vomiting accompanying the headache, prodromal visual phenomena, unilateral pain, and a family history of similar headaches. Although Vahlquist offered no data to establish this definition's statistical validity, his attempt was the first to provide simple criteria for diagnosing the disease.

Bille's (1962) classic study of headache in children attempted to derive empirically the symptoms that were associated with migraines. He examined all 7- to 15-year-old schoolchildren in a moderate-sized Swedish town and obtained a variety of data on the headaches these children experienced. Not surprisingly, the children's headaches fell roughly into two types – tension and migraine. The same four characteristics that Vahlquist (1955) had enumerated were the only ones significantly more frequently associated with migraines than with other headaches. Bille could make an accurate diagnosis in approximately 97% of patients, using the same criteria as Vahlquist had (two of the preceding four characteristics listed plus paroxysmal headache).

The same year (1962), the American Medical Association (AMA) reclassified headaches in both adults and children. Migraine headaches were renamed "vascular headaches" because vascular changes were felt to play a major role in their causation. The AMA listed subgroups within the more general category of migraines. The most important were "classic migraine," which had the characteristic picture of symptoms, and "common migraine," which differed somewhat from the traditional definitions of migraine (e.g., bilateral pain) but still followed the basic pattern of paroxysmal headache. The AMA also defined tension headaches according to their suspected etiology (i.e., as associated with contraction of skeletal muscles).

More recent definitions (e.g., Prensky & Sommer, 1976) have sought to reconcile the AMA model with those of Bille and Vahlquist. These newer definitions cite longer lists of symptoms typically associated with migraine; having paroxysmal headache and a few of the symptoms implies "common migraine," whereas having most or all of the symptoms and paroxysmal headache implies "classic migraine." None of these definitions has addressed the subjective experience of the pain: intensity, duration, interference with daily activities, and so forth.

An additional factor often used to classify migraine headaches is the presence of the "migraine personality." People who suffer from migraine headaches have been said to be anxious, highly motivated towards achievement, above average in intelligence, and often obsessive about completing work and fulfilling responsibilities. However, systematic research (e.g., Bille, 1982) has refuted this contention. The "migraine personality" does not define migraine sufferers; no statistical evidence supports the idea of a specific personality being associated with most or all migraine patients. Although many migraine sufferers do have these personality characteristics, many do not.

Differential Diagnosis

It is often necessary to differentiate a migraine headache from other intracranial processes. Several different conditions can produce symptoms strikingly similar to those of migraine. Cranial tumors, particularly early in their development, can present with a sharp pain of sudden onset, often with periods when the pain remits. Depending on their location, they may be accompanied by sensory auras. In this case, computerized axial tomography (CAT) can identify a tumor mass. Moreover, as a tumor grows, its symptomatic presentation will change and often intensify.

Epilepsy is another disturbance frequently confused with migraine. Rothner (1978) noted that children who have headache associated with sensory auras are often diagnosed as having seizures despite equivocal electroencephalographic (EEG) findings. The two syndromes have similar clinical presentations, frequently involving sensory auras, sudden onset attacks of limited duration, pain, nausea, and vomiting. Moreover, an abnormal EEG does not necessarily either imply the presence of a seizure disorder or rule out migraines. Froelich, Carter, O'Leary, and Rosenbaum (1960) found that of 271 children diagnosed as having migraine but not epilepsy, 51% had abnormal EEGs, many with patterns suggestive of epilepsy. A number of studies (e.g., Millichap, 1978; Ziegler & Wong, 1967) have reached similar conclusions.

The EEGs of many migraine patients are abnormal, but this does not imply that many children who have migraines have seizures or vice versa. Suter, Klingman, Austin, and Lacy (1959) found that only about 4% of children with seizures had migraine headaches. This is far too small a number of account for the vast majority of children with migraine who have abnormal EEGs.

If seizures and migraine headaches can appear to be so similar in children, how may a differential diagnosis be made, particularly if the EEG is not helpful? Brown (1977) cited several differences between the two groups. Compared with children with epilepsy, children with migraines had many more headaches, few or no convulsions, a much greater likelihood of having a family member with migraine, and headaches lasting minutes to hours rather than a few seconds to a few minutes. Jay and Tomasi (1980) found five key symptoms that appeared to be useful in separating the two groups. Unlike migraine sufferers, patients with seizures had impaired consciousness during their headaches, postictal confusion, and a family history of seizures. Their EEGs showed severely abnormal findings, and these patients showed a positive response to anticonvulsant medications.

The differential diagnosis between migraine and tension headache is, in some instances, quite difficult. Although on initial consideration, the two types of headache appear to be so different, one might expect they could hardly be mistaken for each other. Yet some individual's headaches seem to have symptoms of both types. The AMA (1962) called these "combination headaches." Further, common migraine headaches may be bilateral, have no preheadache aura, and may cause neither nausea or vomiting. Severe tension headaches, on the other hand, may sometimes appear to have a unilateral focus and cause nausea and vomiting. Therefore, the line between the two disorders may not be as clear as was first suspected.

Joffe, Bakal, and Kaganov (1983) studied 47 children with intense headache, previously diagnosed as either migraine or tension headache. After 3 weeks, they evaluated whether these patients' symptoms fell into the clusters expected (migraine versus tension) or if there was an overlap between the two groups' symptoms. A mixing of symptoms traditionally identified with the two types of headache was frequent, and few patients had "pure" headaches of either type. They proposed a model of the relationship between the two types of headache, suggesting that migraines and tension headaches occur on a continuum that had 100% migraine headaches at one end and 100% tension headaches at the other. Intermediate values occurred in between.

Also falling on a continuum is the level of organic involvement in the etiology of both migraine and tension headaches. Migraines have been somewhat incorrectly assumed to be entirely "organic" because of their vascular component, and tension headaches were, by their very name, psychogenic. However, some migraine patients have attacks that occur primarily after stressful events, and some patients have tension headaches that do not appear to be related to identifiable psychosocial stressors, but who are found to have significant muscle tension. Etiologic factors appear to fall on a continuum, with "all organic" at one end and "all psychogenic" at the other.

DSM III criteria for conversion disorders excludes this diagnosis in the presence of any pathophysiology, which many of the tension headache patients have, and which is assumed in all migraine patients. Diagnosis of headaches as a psychogenic pain disorder is complicated by the requirement that either no organic pathology be present or that the patient reports pain grossly in excess of the known organic pathology.

Distinguishing headaches that are symptomatic of conversion disorder (or are a psychogenic pain disorder) from migraine is made easier by the temporal association with a precipitating event in conversion. This distinction may not be so clear when differentiating between tension and conversion headache. Many tension headaches, and a few migraine headaches, may also fit DMS III criteria for diagnosis of conversion disorder. Patients present with headaches temporally related to psychosocial stressors. These headaches significantly change the patient's daily activities and the response of significant others to the patient. Finally, the headaches are not under voluntary control. These headaches also are not responsive to treatment with conservative therapies such as analgesics. Other tension and migraine headaches appear to approach the DMS III definition of a psychogenic pain disorder. These patients have some identifiable organic involvement in their pain, yet seen to exaggerate their symptoms, particularly in the presence of stressors.

Another group of patients are seen with headaches as part of a syndrome of multiple complaints involving many bodily areas. These patients most closely resemble the DSM III diagnosis of somatization disorder. Other patients have headaches that are symptomatic of a depressive episode. Such headaches are found to occur only when the patient has a dysphoric mood, low self-esteem, as well as other symptoms of affective disorder including vegetative symptoms.

The importance of a differential diagnosis lies in the implications of a diagnostic label for treatment and prognosis. In the case of tumors or seizures, treatments will likely differ substantially from that which would be given for migraines. In the case of tension headaches, as will be seen, treatments may also differ from that given for migraine, although in a more subtle way. Conversion headaches require similar symptom amelioration, but perhaps more attention to acute and/or chronic psychiatric problems. Therefore, in treating headaches, a correct diagnosis is the first essential task.

Epidemiology of Childhood Headache

What is the prevalence of headache in childhood? Vahlquist (1955) surveyed a large population of children age 10 to 12 years and 16 to 19 years and determined the incidence of either frequent tension headache or migraine headache. He found that in his younger group, almost 5% had migraines and 13% had tension headaches; in the older group, the figures were 7% and 19%, respectively. Vahlquist concluded that headache was a problem for a significant portion of the pediatric population.

Bille (1962) provided the most complete epidemiologic record, having obtained data from well over 95% of 7- to 15-year-olds in the Swedish city of Uppsala. With the results summed across all ages, it was found that 41% had no headaches, 48% had only occasional nonmigrainous headaches, 7% had frequent tension headaches, and 4% had migraine headaches. This last 11% was considered to be the group that might be appropriate for treatment.

Bille also analyzed trends for age and sex. Males generally had more headaches than females until age 10, when females caught up with and then surpassed males, eventually having many more headaches. Except for migraines in males, which leveled off and then dropped somewhat after age 10, the numbers of all types of headaches increased by year for both sexes.

A variety of other epidemiologic studies have been completed since Bille's report, many in Scandinavia. Sillanpaa (1976) performed a study much like Bille's, involving all 7-year-old schoolchildren in a town in Finland. Sillanpaa found that 13% of the 7-year-olds had more than one headache each month, and that 3.2% had migraines; these figures were similar to those of Bille's youngest subjects, who were also 7 years of age.

Sillanpaa (1983) followed up these same children 7 years later; all types of headaches increased significantly. At age 14, almost 75% of these adolescents had headaches at least once a month; 8% of the males and 15% of the females had migraines (11.3% of the population). These frequencies were significantly higher than those in previous reports.

What can we conclude about the epidemiology of headaches? First, they are a significant problem at all ages studied and that the proportion of children affected increases with age. By the late teens, as much as 18% of the population may be afflicted. Also by the late teens, more girls than boys have headaches, including migraines.

Prognosis of Childhood Headache

Several studies have addressed the question of whether children with headaches continue to have these symptoms throughout life. Bille (1973) followed up 73 patients between 4 and 14 years of age after they first sought medical help for their childhood-onset migraines. These patients had received treatment consisting primarily of medication. Fourteen years after initial diagnosis, 41% of the subjects were asymptomatic, 32% were "significantly improved," and only 27% had not improved or were worse.

Sillanpaa (1983) followed a group of children from age 7 to age 14. He found that of those who had had migraines at age 7, 37% were asymptomatic, 22% improved, and 41% the same or worse at age 14. Males and those whose headaches started at younger ages did better. These data are similar to if somewhat less optimistic than Bille's (1973).

Congdon and Forsythe (1979) did a follow-up study specifically designed to evaluate the prognosis of migraine. Three hundred childhood-onset migraine patients were reevaluated 4 to 15 years after their original complaint. Of these, 37% had had a complete remission, but the authors noted that all of these remissions had occurred by age 18; all subjects who had migraines at age 18 continued to have them for the period studied. No data are given for "improvement" without complete remission. However, the 37% figure matches that of Sillanpaa.

Hinrichs and Keith (1965) performed a study worth noting. They followed up 92 children for at least 9 years after the onset of their migraines and found that 81% of males were found to be significantly improved or asymptomatic compared with only 59% of females.

Thus, at least 60% of all patients whose migraines begin in childhood will have significant improvement or remission of symptoms. Males are more likely to have a positive outcome than are females. Some data support the idea that if remission is going to occur, it will occur by age 18 or not at all. The reason for this high remission rate is purely speculative. It may be that the maturation of vascular and neurologic systems plays a role. In the case of tension headaches, older children may cope better and express tension in some way other than through muscular contraction. For conversion headaches, frequent spontaneous improvement has been described; for a somatization disorder, shifting to another physical symptom is common.

The fact that many children have remissions of their headaches does not imply that treatment is unnecessary. Children may suffer with migraines or other headaches for several years before remission. These headaches can significantly impair school and social activities and family relationships. Since in some cases treatment may prevent years of pain and disruption of the child's life, intervention is certainly indicated.

Although the prognostic studies provide firm evidence that many children have a positive outcome, several important issues remain unaddressed. Do variables such as age of onset, frequency of headache, intensity of headache, duration of headaches, and psychological characteristics affect the prognosis? No conclusive data are available. Clearly, more studies are needed to clarify the issue of prognosis for childhood-onset headache.

Treatment of Pediatric Headache

A variety of therapies has been tried both to prevent recurrence and alleviate the symptoms of headache. For mild infrequent headaches, many individuals take nonprescription analgesics. For more severe headaches, a variety of therapies is used. Medication is frequently the first modality. Severe tension headache sufferers are often given antianxiety drugs such as Valium; unfortunately, this has proven to have limited effectiveness, often with significant side effects. Pharmacotherapy for migraine sufferers has also been of limited effectiveness. A variety of medications, involving antidepressants, anticonvulsants, antianxiety drugs, and most often ergotamine-derivatives, has proven highly successful in some cases, but has been of little help in others. More recently, special diets have been tried, particularly involving avoiding caffeine and/or foods that are involved in tyramine synthesis. Although spectacularly successful with some patients, these diets have little use in others.

Psychotherapy has sometimes been useful with both children and adults, relieving the stress that causes anxiety. Often, the general advice to these patients is that they "avoid stress," good advice for almost all people, but in many situations difficult to carry out given the demands of daily living. In our clinical experience, psychotherapy is effective for some headache patients. Children rarely spontaneously make the connection between physical symptoms and psychosocial stress, anxiety, or depression. If the person changes in ways that permit them to live more comfortably with themselves, other stress will naturally decline. If the headache serves a defensive function such as turning a person's anger at another against himself, understanding the symptom's function may reduce the patient's need for it. However, not everyone benefits from psychotherapy.

The greatest success with dynamic psychotherapy has been with children whose verbal skills are good and who have been clearly stressed in the recent past. Apart from conversion disorders, children with tension rather than migraine headaches have benefited most. Psychotherapy is also frequently used with patients who have headaches as symptoms of affective or anxiety disorders. Psychotherapeutic techniques with these patients vary greatly, based on the patient's age, the nature of his or her headache, the stressors, and the psychopathology. To further demonstrate the use of psychotherapy with a headache patient, a case example is presented.

Scott is an 8-year-old boy with high average intelligence and excellent verbal skills, who has suffered from severe headaches for approximately 6 months. Prior to that, Scott suffered only from very mild infrequent headaches. However, he had occasionally seen his father get headaches related to stress that were so severe that the father had to take bed rest for short periods. This symptom attracted a great deal of sympathy from the family. Scott was also aware of a maternal aunt who had migraine headaches that periodically caused her to drop her activities and rest in a dark quiet room.

Scott developed problem headaches shortly after two highly stressful life events. First, a dog who had been in the family ever since Scott could remember and to whom he was very attached was put to sleep against Scott's will. Shortly afterward, Scott's music teacher was murdered in her sleep in a highly publicized case. Following these two events, Scott developed a number of depressive symptoms. He lost his appetite, had trouble sleeping and doing schoolwork, was unhappy, and withdrew socially. Simultaneously, he developed severe headaches, particularly around bedtime, when he refused to go to sleep without a parent present and tried to sleep with his eyes open. Scott almost certainly feared that sleep would lead to death, both as in his dog's being "put to sleep" and as occurring at the time of his teacher's murder.

The evaluator felt that Scott's headaches were part of an acute depressive syndrome related to stressful life events. The headaches were a way to express distress as well as a means to gaining attention and nurturance from his parents, whose physical presence at bedtime was reinforcing.

Scott was then seen for one individual psychotherapy session per week. In this therapy, work was done to help Scott recognize when he was afraid, and he was encouraged to seek out responsible others (parents at home, a social worker at school) when he became afraid, particularly at bedtime. After eight sessions, Scott's headaches remitted and there was improvement in all of his depressive symptoms. He was able to seek out nurturance and support from others and verbally express his fears.

Psychotherapy was chosen as a treatment for Scott because it was felt that his depressive symptoms seemed primary and that the reasons for his headache were clearly linked to the precipitants of his depression and fear. Because psychotherapy helped Scott develop new skills in expressing feelings, the anxiety generated by these precipitants could be resolved. Also, Scott has good resources, which contributed to the success of therapy. Finally, it may well have been that tension was significant in Scott's headaches, but as a direct response to stress. It was felt that teaching Scott to relax those muscles might help end some headaches, but would not address the underlying emotional distress.

Because many migraine and tension headache sufferers were unable to obtain relief through these therapeutic modalities, different treatments were needed. A fortuitous coincidence at Elmer Green's laboratory at the Menninger Foundation led to the development of such a treatment. Green was performing a study in which patients were asked to raise the temperature of their hands by simple concentration and visualization ("handwarming"). One patient spontaneously reported that her handwarming had stopped a migraine headache that was in the prodromal stage. This led to a series of studies designed to determine if handwarming could, indeed, be used to treat migraine headaches.

Three investigators performed the original investigations of the treatment of migraine headache at the Menninger Foundation (Sargent, Green, & Walters, 1972; Sargent, Green, & Walters, 1973a; Sargent, Walters, & Green, 1973b). The paradigm they used involves treating migraines with a combination of relaxation training, "autogenic training" (self-suggestion), and thermal biofeedback, which involved taking the temperature differential between the hand and the forehead. Typically, before biofeedback, the forehead is considerably warmer; after biofeedback, little if any temperature difference can be detected. Patients were asked to keep "headache diaries," which were records of the frequency, intensity, duration, and site of their headaches, to determine if treatment led to any variance in the headaches before and after treatment.

Several theories have been proposed to account for why handwarming would control migraine headaches. In simplest form, training patients to concentrate on warming their hands was hypothesized as increasing blood flow to their extremities while simultaneously decreasing cerebrovascular flow, thereby correcting the vascular problems that cause migraine.

The authors conducted three separate studies. In each, more than 80% of migraine patients had either complete remission of their symptoms or a significant improvement. The best outcomes were found in the youngest patients (younger than 21 years), more than 90% of whom had a successful outcome. This suggested that pediatric patients in particular might benefit from this procedure.

Finally, patients who successfully learned handwarming were almost all in the successful outcome group; those who failed simply did not learn handwarming. The researchers concluded that psychological variables likely prevented the patients from learning the handwarming–in other words, that for unspecified reasons, the patients feared losing their headaches.

Further proof of this procedure's efficacy was found by Solbach and Sargent (1978), who followed up these same patients for a minimum of 2 years after treatment. Subjects who completed treatment as well as those who dropped out were seen at follow-up. Both groups were found to be improved when compared with pretreatment migraine levels. Patients who had completed treatment and were rated immediately posttreatment as having a very good outcome had the best outcome at follow-up. These data provided significant evidence that biofeedback could provide long-term relief from migraines.

Several studies also addressed the efficacy of thermal feedback with patients who had tension headaches and headaches with both tension and migraine components. In general, these patients have not done as well with the thermal feedback (e.g., Fahrion, 1977; Fried, Lamberti, & Sneed, 1977).

Simply put, thermal biofeedback should not have been expected to prove as successful with combination and tension headache patients since migraine is believed to be rooted in vascular changes; tension headache is related to muscle tension in the shoulder, neck, and head muscles. Tension in these muscles is better measured using electrical conductance across the muscle at any given time; in general, the higher the current, the more serious the tension. Therefore, investigators interested in treating tension headaches with biofeedback looked to measuring and reducing muscle contractions. Electromyelography (EMG), which measures such current, was an excellent tool.

Budzynski, Stoyva, Adler, and Mullaney (1973) performed the seminal study of biofeedback treatment of tension headache. They studied 36 adults with tension headaches, divided into three groups: (a) those receiving true EMG biofeedback, (b) those receiving false EMG biofeedback, and (c) controls receiving treatment. Patients in the first group were expected to be the only ones who would improve. Since only they had accurate feedback on tension in their forehead, no one else really would know when such tension was being decreased.

The study confirmed the hypothesis. Only the patients in the first group had significant decreases in the frequency, intensity, and duration of their tension headaches. Neither of the other two groups differed significantly from their prestudy status, ruling out a placebo effect. What further indicated the efficacy of this treatment was the observation that when accurate biofeedback was then given to the second and third groups, each group improved significantly. Numerous replications of this study have yielded amost uniformly positive results (Diamond & Montrose, 1984; Wickramasekera, 1972).

Unfortunately, these studies were done with all or nearly all adult subjects. Werder and Sargent (1984) did a study that examined the efficacy of biofeedback in treating children with headaches. They examined patients with three types of headaches (migraine, tension, and combination). Migraine patients were treated with thermal biofeedback; combination and tension patients were given EMG biofeedback. Werder and Sargent then followed up these patients for 2 to 3 years after they completed treatment. Ninety percent of the patients were said to have successful outcomes at the end of formal biofeedback treatment (i.e., a reduction of 51% or more in frequency, intensity, and duration of headaches) and 60% of them were found to have maintained these gains 2 to 3 years later. On the whole, the results of the studies are convincing. Despite some methodological flaws, the weight of evidence supports the notion that children with headaches are excellent candidates for treatment with biofeedback and that biofeedback can provide significant long-term relief for sufferers of migraine, tension, and combination headaches.

To further demonstrate a standard technique of biofeedback for headache, a case example is presented. It involves a girl with an unusually mixed presentation.

Susan is a 12-year-old female with superior-range intelligence, who has suffered from severe headaches since she was 2-years-old. Initially, most of these headaches were tension headaches, occurring approximately one or two times per month, and relieved fairly well with over-the-counter analgesics. Once or twice a year, Susan developed migraine-like headaches that forced her to go to bed and rest; the bedrest typically resolved these headaches. However, in the year before she entered treatment, Susan's migraines dramatically increased in frequency, intensity, and duration. They began to occur once every 2 to 3 weeks and required long periods of bedrest and sleep before resolving. The migraine headaches typically began with a visual aura involving bright lights, nausea, and vomiting; they then progressed to a headache phase involving severe pain, which forced the patient to discontinue whatever activity she was involved in and seek bedrest. The patient's family history is positive for migraines.

Susan was seen by a neurologist, who referred the patient for biofeedback and suggested that she keep an informal headache record before her first biofeedback session. This first session was approximately 1 month after the patient's neurologic evaluation, and this interval served as the baseline period. Susan's headache diary revealed two migraine and two tension headaches during this period.

The first choice to be made by the therapist was what type of biofeedback the patient should receive. Unlike patients with combination headaches, who have symptoms of migraine and tension headaches at the same time, Susan had separate headaches that appeared to be either entirely tension headaches or entirely migraine headaches. There was no combination of symptoms during any one headache. It was decided that the patient should have thermal biofeedback because it was the migraines that had increased in severity and led to her seeking medical/psychological treatment.

During the first session, a brief informal explanation was given as to the reason that she was receiving biofeedback; this explanation involved discussion of the presence of vascular changes in migraine headaches and the fact that handwarming represented self-regulation of blood vessels. Following this explanation, Susan was given several autogenic phrases to concentrate on, focusing on relaxing her muscles and feeling warmth in her hands.

After this, the first training session began. A temperature probe was attached to Susan's right index finger, and she was placed in front of a video monitor that displayed a bar graph representing the temperature of her finger. She was asked to concentrate on feeling relaxed and imagining warmth flowing into her hands. She almost immediately displayed excellent control of her hand temperature, and she was able to elevate the temperature in her hands by several degrees during the first session. Following six 3-minute trials, the biofeedback was concluded for the session, which then ended with a brief discussion of biofeedback. Susan was also asked to practice handwarming at home, twice each day for 15 minutes per session.

The second formal training session occurred 4 days after the first. Susan reported having had no headaches in the interim, and had complied with the daily practice regimen. During the second session, she was given a brief period to concentrate on autogenic relaxation and handwarming phrases, and then was given six 3-minute thermal biofeedback trials. Susan again displayed excellent biofeedback control and was able to relate the temperature in her hands to the subject she was thinking about (e.g., high hand temperature when concentrating on handwarming, low hand temperature when thinking about family fights). The session concluded with a discussion period, and Susan was instructed to maintain the same home practice regimen.

Five more training sessions were conducted, with a 1-week interval between sessions. The sessions were conducted at weekly intervals because this was the most practical alternative for Susan, and because she demonstrated such excellent command of handwarming procedures. During these 5 weeks, Susan only experienced one mild headache, and she related this to not having eaten for an extended period; this headache was resolved by her eating dinner.

A 3-month follow-up was conducted. During that time, she had practiced relaxation and handwarming approximately once per day. She reported having had only one mild tension headache, which quickly resolved with aspirin. There had been no recurrence of migraine headaches.

Several points are noteworthy in this case. First, as frequently happens in a clinical setting, the patient presented with symptoms that differed from those reported in the research literature. Clinicians must determine what intervention is appropriate based on the presenting symptom picture. Next, treatment occurred at longer intervals and for fewer sessions than is typical in research protocols. However, practical considerations and the patient's rapid acquisition of handwarming and relaxation skills made this a viable alternative.

Finally, the effect of thermal biofeedback was striking on both the migraine and the tension headaches. Perhaps the relaxation associated with handwarming decreased the muscle tension in the patient's neck and scalp and accounted for the decrease in tension headaches. Also, returning a sense of control to the child may have helped her feel less stress and tension.

Summary

Headaches are afflictions that interfere to varying degrees with the lives of the vast majority of the population. Children are not excluded. Headaches can be caused by physiologic and psychological factors and combinations thereof. A variety of treatments has proven to be of limited success in alleviating the pain of the various types of headaches. Medication, psychotherapy, and biofeedback all play an important role in the successful treatment of headaches in childhood.

References

American Medical Association, Ad Hoc Committee on Classification of Headache. (1962). Classification of headache. *Journal of the American Medical Association*, *179*, 717-718.

Apley, J. (1975). *The child with abdominal pain*. Oxford: Blackwell Scientific Publications.

Bille, B. (1962). Migraine in school children. *Acta Paediatrica Scandinavica*, (*Suppl. 136*), 1-152.

Bille, B., (1973). The prognosis of migraine in childhood. *Acta Paediatrica Scandinavica*, (*Suppl. 236*), 38.

Brown, J.K. (1977). Migraine and migraine equivalents in children. *Developmental Medicine and Child Neurology*, *19*, 683-692.

Budzinski, T.H., Stoyva, J., Adler, C., & Mullaney, D. (1973). EMG biofeedback and tension headache: A controlled outcome study. *Psychosomatic Medicine*, *35*, 484-496.

Christensen, M.F., & Mortenson, O. (1975). Long-term prognosis in children with recurrent abdominal pain. *Archives of Diseases of Childhood*, *50*, 110-114.

Congdon, P., & Forsythe, W. (1979). Migraine in childhood: A study of 300 children. *Developmental medicine and child neurology*, *21*, 209-216.

Diamond, S., & Montrose, D. (1984). The value of biofeedback in the treatment of chronic headache: A four-year retrospective study. *Headache*, *24*, 5-18.

Fahrion, S. (1977). Autogenic biofeedback treatment for migraine. *Mayo Clinic Proceedings*, *52*, 776-784.

Farrell, M.K. (1984). Abdominal pain. *Pediatrics*, *74*(suppl), 955-957.

Fried, F., Lamberti, J., & Sneed, P. (1977). Treatment of tension and migraine headaches with biofeedback techniques. *Missouri Medicine*, *74*, 252-255.

Froelich, W., Carter, C., O'Leary, J., & Rosenbaum, H. (1960). Headache in children: Electroencephalographic evaluation of 500 cases. *Neurology*, *10*, 639-642.

Hinrichs, W., & Keith, H. (1965). Migraine in childhood: A follow-up report. *Mayo Clinic Proceedings*, *40*, 593-596.

Jay, G., & Tomasi, L. (1980). Pediatric headaches: A one-year retrospective analysis. *Headache*, *20*, 5-9.

Joffe, R., Bakal, D., & Kaganov, J. (1983). A self-observation study of headache in childhood. *Headache*, *23*, 20-25.

Millichap, J. (1978). Recurrent headaches in 100 children. *Child's Brain*, *4*, 95-105.

Oster, J. (1972). Recurrent abdominal pain, headache, and limb pains in children and adolescents. *Pediatrics*, *50*, 429-436.

Prensky, A.L., & Sommer, D. (1976). Migraine and migrainous variants in pediatric patients. *Symposium or Pediatric Neurology*, *23*, 461-471.

Rothner, A.D. (1978). Headache in children: A review. *Headache*, *18*, 169-175.

Sargent, J., Green, E., & Walters, M. (1972). The use of autogenic feedback training in a pilot study of migraine and tension headaches. *Headache*, *12*, 120-124.

Sargent, J., Green, E., & Walters, M. (1973a). Preliminary report on the use of autogenic feedback training in the treatment of migraine and tension headaches. *Psychosomatic Medicine*, *35*, 129-135.

Sargent, J., Walters, M., & Green, E. (1973b). Psychosomatic self-regulation of migraine headaches. *Seminars in Psychiatry*, *5*, 415-428.

Sillanpaa, M. (1976). Prevalence of migraine and other headache in Finnish children starting school. *Headache*, *15*, 288-290.

Sillanpaa, M. (1983). Prevalence of migraine and other headaches during the first seven school years. *Headache*, *23*, 15–19.

Solbach, P., & Sargent, J. (1978). A follow-up evaluation of the Menninger Pilot Migraine Study using thermal training. *Headache*, *18*, 198–202.

Stone, R.T., & Barbero, G.J. (1970). Recurrent abdominal pain in childhood. *Pediatrics*, *45*, 732–738.

Suter, C., Klingman, W., Austin, H., & Lacy, O. (1959). Migraine and seizure states in children. *Diseases of the Nervous System*, *20*, 9–16.

Vahlquist, B. (1955). Migraine in children. *International Archives of Allergy*, *7*, 348–355.

Werder, D., & Sargent, J. (1984). A study of childhood headache using biofeedback as a treatment alternative. *Headache*, *24*, 122–126.

Wickramasekera, I. (1972). Electromyographic feedback training and tension headache: Preliminary observations. *American Journal of Clinical Hypnosis*, *15*, 83–85.

Ziegler, D., & Wong, G. (1967). Migraine in children and electroencephalographic studies of families. *Epilepsia*, *8*, 171–187.

9

Pseudoseizures in Children and Adolescents

The type of conversion symptom most frequently reported in the literature and the presenting symptom seen most frequently by physicians is the pseudoseizure, also referred to as a psychogenic or hysterical seizure. These seizure-like phenomena occur without any identifiable cerebral disturbance. Since they are a type of conversion symptom, pseudoseizures can be classified in DSM III as either a conversion disorder or as a feature of a somatization disorder.

Considerable evidence has been gathered that suggests that psychological factors play an important role in pseudoseizures. For example, Gross and Huerta (1980) found evidence of important conflicts in 17 of their 19 cases. Gross and Huerta and others report that the significant types of conflicts or stressors include sexual trauma or abuse, unresolved grief reactions, parental conflict, anxiety over separation from family, learning disability (Silver, 1982), poor performance at school, and poor relations with peers (Williams, Spiegel, & Mostofsky, 1978). Anticonvulsant medications, which often appear to have detrimental effects on cognition and emotional states (Trimble, 1982), may also be a precipitating factor (Niedermeyer, Blumer, Holscher, & Walker, 1970). Many reports note that families may provide patients with pseudoseizure with secondary gain in the form of extra attention and special considerations. Williams et al. (1978) and Holmes, Sackellares, McKiernan, Ragland, & Dreifuss (1980) noted that the frequency of pseudoseizures decreased dramatically purely in response to psychological interventions. Holmes et al. (1980) also reported that these patients usually do not respond to changes in medication, while pseudoseizures increase in frequency when these patients are stressed. Finlayson and Lucas (1979) compared the Minnesota Multiphasic Personality Inventory (MMPI) profiles of pseudoseizure patients with those of a group of adolescents receiving medical care for other reasons, and found more evidence of nonspecific psychopathology in the pseudoseizure group. Of the five cases of pseudoseizures Goodyer (1985) reported, none had personality disorders or depression, but anxiety was a frequent psychological concomitant.

Although most pseudoseizures appear to serve as an indirect way of expressing

---

This chapter was written with Bruce Renken.

anxiety or gaining attention, these patients do not seem to have voluntary control over their seizures. Because no one knows how the underlying psychological factors are translated into involuntary symptoms that simulate neurologic ones, it is difficult to delineate precisely which psychological processes are relevant to pseudoseizures.

Pseudoseizures were recorded in ancient literature and were described in detail in the late nineteenth century, most notably by Gowers (Massey, 1982). Modern medical and psychiatric literature generally ignored them. However, since Bernstein (1969) reported several cases of pseudoseizures in adolescent girls experiencing sexual pressures, a considerable number of cases of both children and adults have appeared in the literature.

Increased interest in pseudoseizures is due to the increasing evidence that sexual abuse or sexual trauma is an important etiologic factor in pseudoseizures. As was pointed out in Chapter 1, there is a renewed interest in the relationship between sexual trauma in childhood and the later development of psychopathology—a relationship that formed the basis of Freud's work but, that until recently was ignored by much of the academic world (Masson, 1985; Rosenfeld, 1979; Rosenfeld, Nadelson, & Krieger, 1979). Pseudoseizures are the conversion symptom that provided some of the clearest documentation of this relationship.

Several reports have appeared of small selected samples of adolescent females whose pseudoseizures appear to be related to sexual trauma. Bernstein (1969), Goodwin, Simms, and Bergman (1979), Gross (1979), and LaBarbera and Dozier (1980) described a total of 17 such cases whose symptoms included fainting or falling, rapid shaking, violent thrashing, and coital movements or pelvic jerking with no incontinence. Although most of the other cases involved little or no loss of consciousness, Gross reports two cases of prolonged absence spells.

The interest in pseudoseizures has also grown, however, because the technique of simultaneous electroencephalographic (EEG) monitoring and video recording of patients with seizures was developed for use in specialized epilepsy treatment centers. Since the seizure is simultaneously recorded on video and on EEG, the events occurring in seizures can be recorded more precisely and detailed distinctions can be made between pseudoseizures and epileptic seizures. This technique has revealed that pseudoseizures are far more frequent among epilepsy patients than was previously suspected. This technique is now considered the most accurate way to diagnose pseudoseizures.

Epidemiology and Symptom Description

Table 9.1 summarizes the finding of a number of studies of the age and sex distribution and associated characteristics of adult pseudoseizure patients (studies of adults are reported because this type of data is extremely scarce for children and adolescents patients). Table 9.2 summarizes the findings of several reports of samples of children and adolescents with pseudoseizures.

As Table 9.1 shows, no generally accepted estimate is available for the incidence of pseudoseizures in the population. Guze, Woodruff, and Clayton (1971)

TABLE 9.1. Selected Findings for Pseudoseizures in Adults

Study	No.	% Female	% with Epilepsy	% with Organic Brain Dysfunction
Krumholtz & Niedermeyer (1983)	41	79	37	44
Cohen & Suter (1982)	51	78	11.8	23.6
Roy (1979)	22	95.6	36.4	NA
Roy (1977)	34	85.3	32.4	38.2
Standage (1975)	25	84	16	32

NA = not available.

found that 1.6% of adult psychiatric outpatients had pseudoseizures. Five to 10% of adults with conversion symptoms are estimated to have pseudoseizures, although Ljungberg (1957) found that 19.9% of patients with conversion symptoms had pseudoseizures as their major symptom, and 35.7% had them as one of their symptoms. However, Ljungberg's study was done in Sweden, which may reflect a different cultural pattern. In addition, Ljungberg based his findings on a complete search of Sweden's national records, whereas the American studies were of more restricted populations. Even less information is available about the incidence of pseudoseizures in children and adolescents. Schneider and Rice (1979) found that pseudoseizures occurred in 25% of children with conversion symptoms (with a total number of only 32), whereas in Maloney's (1980) study (n = 105), the incidence was 7.6%.

Females outnumber males in all samples. For instance, the two random series of child and adolescent pseudoseizure cases included 22 females and 8 males (Holmes et al., 1980; Gross & Huerta, 1980). Although systematic evidence of age differences has not been reported, the literature suggests that pseudoseizures are more common in adolescence than in childhood, and that as in most other somatoform symptoms the sex ratio, which is relatively even in childhood, becomes heavily weighted in favor of females during adolescence.

Pseudoseizures seem to be able to manifest virtually all the behavioral symptoms that characterize epileptic seizures, namely, loss of consciousness, the clonic movements of grand mal seizures, more specific motor behaviors typical of partial complex seizures, fainting, headache, confusion, self-injury, and (according to at least one report) incontinence. Holmes et al. (1980) and Gross and Huerta (1980), drawing cases from specialized epilepsy treatment centers, and Finlayson and Lucas (1979), drawing cases from a general medical facility, compiled information on a total of 48 children and adolescents with pseudoseizures. They found that motor convulsions that resemble either generalized tonic/clonic or partial complex seizures are the most common type of pseudoseizure. "Absence" pseudoseizures (passing out without associated motor disturbance) are apparently less common; Gross and Huerta (1980) found this type of pseudoseizure in only two patients. Motor disturbance in pseudoseizures often involved combativeness, yelling, and crying (Holmes et al., 1980). While consciousness is often altered, in many cases, the patient may be unreponsive only to

TABLE 9.2. Reports of Pseudoseizures in Children and Adolescents

Report	No.	Female/Male Ratio	Major Findings
Samples from specialized epilepsy centers			
Gross & Huerta (1980)[a]	19	14:5	Psychosocial stressors in 17 cases: sexual abuse in 2, overprotective and strict parents in 5, low IQ and academic failure in 2, recent divorce of parents in 4, psychosis in 3. All free of seizures after 1–3 months of treatment.
Holmes et al. (1980)	11	8:3	Eight (72.7%) with both pseudoseizures and epileptic seizures. Predominance of tonic/clonic and partial complex pseudoseizures. No absence pseudoseizures. Combativeness, crying yelling, and vulgar language in pseudoseizures, but not in epileptic seizures.
Williams et al. (1978)	6	4:2	Psychotherapy successful in all cases without definite differential diagnosis. One year follow-up: 4 seizure-free, 2 with fewer seizures.
Adolescent females with histories of sexual abuse			
LaBarbera & Dozier (1980)	4		Sexual conflict in all cases. Sexual trauma precipitating first seizure. Sexual precipitants for later seizures.
Gross (1979a)	4		Two with epilepsy. All with rape in previous 2 years. Three with suicide attempts.
Goodwin et al. (1979)	6		All incest victims. Some with epilepsy, but developed pseudoseizures after incest. Three with suicide attempts or threats.
Bernstein (1969)	3		All with sexual pressures; 1 with abuse. Immature personality development. Alleviation of symptoms with removal of pressures.
Other studies of children with pseudoseizures			
Goodyer (1985)	5	3:2	Epilepsy in 2. No evidence of personality disorder or depression. Conversion in 2, Briquet's in 1, and anxiety neurosis in 1.

TABLE 9.2. *Continued*

Report	No.	Female/Male Ratio	Major Findings
Finlayson & Lucas (1979)[a]	18	11:7	Limited alteration of consciousness, motor symptoms, headache, and hyperventilation common. Abnormal MMPIs. History of extensive diagnostic procedures.
Schneider & Rice (1979)[b]	8	6:2	Pseudoseizures stopped with psychotherapy in 7. At least 1 incest victim.

[a] Patients with epileptic seizures were excluded.
[b] Subgroup from a study of children with conversion disorders.

verbal stimuli (Finlayson & Lucas, 1979). Self-injury and a postictal state of confusion or lethargy are rare, although Holmes et al. (1980) observed the state in some cases. Finlayson and Lucas (1979) found that hyperventilation and headaches were frequently associated with the pseudoseizures. Only one case of incontinence has been found (Scott, 1982).

Subtypes of Pseudoseizures

As the information available about pseudoseizures increases, the question arises as to whether more than one type of pseudoseizure exists. A careful reading of reported cases, our own clinical experiences, and knowledge of conversion symptoms in general suggest that subcategories of pseudoseizures can be identified, with different patterns of symptoms as well as probable differences in etiology and prognosis. Ramani (personal communication, May 1985) has suggested that three types of pseudoseizures can be identified: (a) a type that coexists with epilepsy, (b) an acute conversion type, and (c) a type associated with a chronic, polysymptomatic presentation. The categorization we propose may be influenced by current trends in reporting. However, while other categorizations are possible, we feel that this classification points to some obvious distinctions and allows a clearer presentation of the relationships among etiology, symptoms, and treatment. Goodyer (1985) reported that two of five cases of pseudoseizures had a monosymptomatic disorder (conversion), and one of five had a polysymptomatic disorder.

The first type of pseudoseizure occurs in individuals who have also had epileptic seizures and generally begin after the seizures have been brought under control. Many of these patients have known brain damage and are often mentally retarded. In these patients, the pseudoseizures and secondary gain are usually clearly related. They enact a particular social role, namely, that of the epileptic with a chronic illness to draw attention to themselves. Only after the epileptic seizures have been brought under control do the pseudoseizures begin.

Charles is a 16-year-old mildly retarded boy whose generalized seizures were under control with Depakene until he was moved to a new high school so he could obtain vocational training. Soon after the transfer, he developed sudden akinetic attacks. He would collapse onto the floor and lie there for a period of time. He would then be able to sit and only later would resume normal activities. The spells occurred in very specific situations: when entering a room, going into a new situation, or getting on the school bus.

Two psychological factors appeared to be operating. First, Charles identified himself as an epileptic. He willingly told any interviewer about his seizures and the medication he took. He even appeared to take pride in his condition. Second, Charles had a history of rituals and phobias. Part of his anxiety over adjusting to the new school became evident in his reluctance to get on the bus, enter the school, move from one class to another, and meet new peers. His anxiety in these situations bordered on panic and appeared to contribute to his akinetic attacks. The attention that he obtained from peers and teachers also reinforced these symptoms.

Treatment for Charles involved direct suggestion that he would be able to overcome these symptoms. In addition, positive reinforcement was given when he was able to accomplish a previously avoided behavior without an akinetic attack. Simultaneously, the symptom was ignored; his attacks became less frequent. Also, Charles was put into a group with other adolescents with epilepsy to enable him to make friends and identify as an epileptic without having the pseudoseizures.

The second type, the acute conversion pseudoseizure, is most frequently seen in adolescent females. Although these seizures are commonly associated with sexual trauma, they occasionally are seen in adolescents with other crises. These individuals respond to psychological intervention and quickly give up their symptoms if therapeutic support follows an explicit statement of their symptoms' nature. These individuals also appear to have a high incidence of depression and frequently make suicidal threats (Gross, 1979; Goodwin et al., 1979).

Barbara is a 14-year-old girl initially seen for neurologic consultation regarding possible seizures. She developed the signs and symptoms of meningoencephalitis 2½ years previously, and the diagnosis was confirmed by lumbar puncture. She recovered completely, but a year ago her symptoms recurred. Reevaluation revealed no medical problems. Shortly thereafter, Barbara had the first of a series of stereotyped spells, each precipitated by a mild blow on the occiput. A typical spell started with falling to the floor and then jerking the arms and legs for 45 minutes. She had no cyanosis, pallor, incontinence or tongue biting. Barbara would sleep thereafter for 4 to 6 hours and would be perfectly normal afterwards. All medical tests including computed tomography and EEG were normal, except for a slight hyperreflexia on the right side of the body. A trial on Dilantin prescribed by the referring doctor was unsuccessful. Video monitoring during an episode precipitated by a light blow to the occiput revealed no EEG abnormalities.

Barbara's family is best termed "chaotic." Her father is an unemployed treated alcoholic, now on worker's compensation. He talks incessantly about his own physical problems and is very involved in Barbara's physical symptoms. Her mother is a factory worker who is quiet and withdrawn. Six siblings include an older brother also on worker's compensation, an older sister who has been suicidally depressed, a married old brother with brain damage, a 17-year-old sister, a 10-year-old brother, and an 8-year-old sister described as upset about the family problems. All of these people are living in the same household, which Barbara describes as chaotic.

Barbara is a pretty, well groomed, mature-looking adolescent with an excellent school record. She considers her father overprotective and says he is too involved in her symptoms. She describes her mother as painfully shy and unable to stand up to her dominant father. Barbara demonstrates little concern about her seizures and describes herself as anxious about her family, but not about herself.

Barbara's psychological testing revealed that her intelligence and achievement were average. Her memory and visual motor coordination were good, but she was inattentive to detail. Personality assessment suggested that although Barbara's resources are good, she blocks her emotional response to affective stimuli. A large number of internal and external stressors are present. Barbara's only defenses against them are denial and repression. She is concerned about her sexuality, avoids negative affect, and has an inordinate need to be "good." Mild depression and anxiety were noted as was passivity in the face of stress.

The evaluator felt that Barbara had a conversion reaction that was precipitated by family stress. Although sexual abuse or overstimulation were suspected as having played a role, Barbara denied any sexual activity. When the cause of the seizures was explained to her, Barbara was motivated to try psychotherapy; her father, however, was not convinced. Barbara attended three sessions of psychotherapy. When her father decided that because she no longer had seizures, he would no longer cooperate, therapy was terminated. Despite this, Barbara continued to see the school psychologist, to whom the primary responsibility for the case was transferred.

Pseudoseizure associated with a chronic polysymptomatic disorder is the third type. Individuals with this ailment, usually adolescent females, appear to have been or are at risk for developing somatization disorder (Briquet's syndrome). They often have demanding, dependent personalities, which makes these patients difficult to manage in clinical settings. They come from families that often use psychosomatic symptoms to communicate basic needs. As a rule, these patients have multiple symptoms and a changing symptom pattern. The pseudoseizures may cease, only to recur or have a different symptom replace it. Unfortunately, these adolescents seem to have a poor prognosis for recovery.

David is a 13-year-old eighth grader who was hospitalized on the inpatient pediatric neurology service in March for evaluation of multiple physical complaints, which included dizziness, headaches, vomiting, "hot and cold flashes," "blind spells," and excessive sleepiness. He has not been to school for the past 3 months because he has had one motor seizure a day. David has been receiving special education in English (primarily reading). When he was 3, David had California encephalitis, and since then has had generalized motor seizures and mild choreiform movements. The seizures had been well controlled on Tegretol and Zarontin. During the hospitalization, the staff observed no seizures. No medical cause was found for David's symptoms.

During the diagnostic workup, David was demanding and mildly provocative. He asked to be taken from the ward to the clinic in a wheelchair. During the interview, he seemed to enjoy describing his somatic complaints. He stated that he often would rather stay home than go to school because the teachers were so critical of him. He often feels that other students leave him out and tease him. Since he has been staying home, he sleeps until noon and watches soap operas on TV with his mother. He often sleeps 16 hours a day. He has seen no friends for the past 3 months.

Family history reveals that for the past year, David's father has been disabled as a result of a work injury. His mother, a highly anxious woman, describes David as sickly. During the interview, she focused on David's physical symptoms and on the failure of medical treatment to control his somatic complaints. She complains that his seizures are recurrent and the side effects from anticonvulsant medications are multiple. She describes her relationship to David as close and says that David is unable to provide care for himself because he has numerous falls as a result of his physical weakness. Therefore, she must provide close supervision to protect him from serious injury.

There are six other siblings, all but one older than David. They all live in close proximity to the family home. The mother describes herself as close to all the siblings, including the married ones, and influential in their lives. According to the social worker who interviewed the parents, the family was unsophisticated and inarticulate; their family system was enmeshed.

On psychological testing, David had very slow reaction times. He often arrived at the correct answer long after the question had been asked. Toward the end of the testing, he began to complain, showed decreased effort, and attempted to manipulate the examiner into ending the testing. David has average intelligence, with even performance except in those tests measuring short-term auditory memory and visual motor skills. He was also noted to have difficulty with attention. His achievement was poor in all areas except for reading. Written language was most difficult for him. Personality evaluation revealed a markedly dependent behavior pattern. David is preoccupied with bodily complaints, which he uses to avoid frustration and social isolation at school. He perceives his home as nurturing and attentive to his somatic symptoms. Examiners noted that he was mildly depressed.

David was diagnosed as having a somatization disorder along with his seizure disorder. His current pseudoseizures developed out of a long history of secondary gain associated with his seizure disorder. The pseudoseizures are just one of a myriad of physical complaints that serve to avoid school stress, to gain nurturance at home, and meet his dependency needs.

The staff recommended that he return to school immediately, and that he and his parents be involved in psychotherapy. Special education was recommended in written language rather than reading since his reading was far better than his written language skills. The parents followed the recommendation that David return to school immediately and that David's educational program be changed. However, they did not follow through on the psychotherapy until they received the same opinion at another medical center.

Pseudoseizures and Epileptic Seizures: Diagnosis

In some cases, distinguishing between pseudoseizures and epileptic seizures may be relatively easy, especially where secondary gain is clearly making a substantial contribution. The features of pseudoseizures summarized in the previous section, observed directly or by verbal report, are the basis of diagnosis. If the seizures have several of these characteristics (e.g., the patient is only partial unresponsive, the seizures are directly correlated with stress, and there is no postictal lethargy or confusion), the clinician should at least suspect a psychogenic explanation. Tables have been prepared (e.g., Nicoll, 1981; Holmes et al., 1980), which compare the likelihood of specific symptoms and associated features in pseudoseizures and epileptic seizures. However, attempts to identify specific criteria that differentiate definitively between pseudoseizures and epileptic seizures have usually been thwarted: Exceptions are always discovered. For example, Scott (1982) pointed out that limb movements in pseudoseizures are likely to have a "semi-purposeful" character, involving kicking or hitting, while true clonic movements of a grand mal epileptic seizure involve jerking with a changing rhythm. However, this is not a complete distinction. Some partial complex epileptic seizures may involve automatisms, which are more difficult to distinguish from pseudoseizure movement.

Vigorous side to side head movements (as contrasted to unilateral movements in epileptic seizures), "out of phase" arm and leg movements, severe arching of the back, and pelvic thrusting are characteristics of pseudoseizures described by Ramani (personal communication, May 1985) and others.

Other behavioral characteristics that may distinguish between the two kinds of seizures include incontinence (usually absent in pseudoseizures), plantar reflexes (flexor in pseudoseizures), and corneal reflexes (unchanged in pseudoseizures) (Williams & Mostofsky, 1982). Epileptic seizures usually occupy discrete, relatively brief time periods (except status epilepticus), with rapid onset and ending, whereas pseudoseizures often have a more gradual course. In distinguishing between prolonged status epilepticus and pseudoseizures, Scott (1982) noted that status epilepticus, unlike pseudoseizures, is likely to render the patient incoherent. On the other hand, pseudoseizures are less likely to occur when the individual is alone, although exceptions do exist (Scott, 1982). Similarly, two traditional distinguishing features, tongue biting and more general forms of self-injury, do not always distinguish the two types of seizures (Scott, 1982; Holmes et al., 1980).

Interictal EEGs are often used in making the diagnosis of pseudoseizures; however, many problems confound interpretation. Normal EEGs may include features closely resembling epileptiform patterns (Scott, 1982), and mild abnormalities may exist that do not indicate epilepsy. Mildly abnormal EEGs are also common in childhood. Clinicians who do not appreciate this fact frequently misdiagnose epilepsy on the strength of nonspecific EEG abnormalities and seizure-like behavior. A further complication is that in some patients, anticonvulsant medications may produce mild EEG abnormalities (Niedermeyer et al., 1970) that seem to confirm the erroneous diagnosis of epilepsy. On the other hand, a normal EEG does not always rule out seizures. If a patient is taking anticonvulsant medication and has a normal EEG, the medication must be withdrawn to see whether epileptiform patterns will emerge. Some cases of epilepsy produce normal surface EEGs; only depth recording picks up epileptiform activity in these cases (Holmes et al., 1980).

Despite these pitfalls, the interictal EEG may still provide useful information. If the clinician is familiar with the alternate causes of EEG abnormalities and is able to examine the patient's past EEGs, the EEG is more likely to be read accurately. Also, Scott (1982) noted the importance of comparing the amount of epileptiform activity on the EEG with the frequency and severity of the seizure activity that the patient reports. This comparison can help to identify the patient who has both kinds of seizures.

More telling than the interictal EEG is the EEG record of the seizure itself. Simultaneous EEG telemetry and video recording is the most recent advance in technique. A video picture of the patient is displayed on half of a split-screen TV and the simultaneous EEG record on the other. By making recordings over long periods of time, the diagnostician can identify exactly the EEG state at the time of the seizure. Epileptic seizures register on the electroencephalogram in patterns that are distinct from any EEG activity likely to be produced by a pseudoseizure. Epileptic seizures usually involve attenuation of alpha rhythm preceding the seizure, and a flattening of background elements after the seizure, followed by prolonged slowing. In pseudoseizures, a normal alpha rhythm exists immediately before and after the seizure. During the seizure itself, epileptic seizures are characterized by rhythmic spiking, whereas pseudoseizures usually produce nonrhythmic bursts of muscle artifact. Because the muscle artifact often obscures the record during either type of seizure, the most reliable indicators of a pseudoseizure are the normal alpha pattern and the absence of postictal slowing. Scott (1982) provided a detailed account of EEG aspects of epileptic seizures and pseudoseizures.

Two other techniques have been used to discriminate epileptic seizures from pseudoseizures. Serum prolactin levels increase after generalized tonic/clonic epileptic seizures, but not after pseudoseizures. However, they may not increase after partial complex or other epileptic seizures involving limited motor symptoms (Trimble, 1978). Hypnotic induction of seizures reveals several differences between pseudoseizures and epileptic seizures. Pseudoseizures occurring under hypnosis, unlike epileptic seizures, involve no loss of later recall of the seizure, involve no EEG changes, and may be stopped by suggestion (Konikow, 1983).

In trying to distinguish epileptic seizures from pseudoseizures, particularly when telemetered EEG and video recordings are not available, the best procedure seems to be to gather as much evidence as possible and assess the evidence as a whole. For example, the findings of Holmes et al. (1980) suggest that a postictal state of confusion or lethargy rarely occurs in pseudoseizures, but if it does, it is more likely to accompany a pseudoseizure of the grand mal type. It is also important to determine from the clinical evidence in each case whether positive criteria for a conversion disorder are met. Using psychological criteria to establish the diagnosis, rather than relying solely on the absence of neurologic findings, can prevent unnecessary and dangerous medical diagnostic and treatment procedures (Dubowitz & Hersov, 1976; Friedman, 1973). Positive criteria for a conversion disorder include an increase in seizure activity in response to stress and a decrease in response to psychological intervention. However, these are not definitive since they also occur with some epileptic seizures (Williams et al., 1978). As previously discussed, other criteria may include sexual trauma, a change in the character of the seizures with anticonvulsant drug treatment

(Goodwin et al., 1979; Trimble, 1982), and evidence of psychopathology in the individual or the family (Finlayson & Lucas, 1979).

Etiologic Factors

Epilepsy and Organic Deficits

For a subgroup of pseudoseizure patients, epilepsy and pseudoseizures are clearly related. This relationship can be assessed in two ways: by estimating the number of pseudoseizure patients who have epilepsy, or by estimating the number of epileptics who have pseudoseizures.

Table 9.1 suggests that between 10 and 35% of adults with pseudoseizures also have epilepsy. In the report by Holmes et al. (1980) of 11 children with pseudoseizures, 8 (72%) had epilepsy. However, these reports may reflect biases according to the type of population from which they were drawn. Specialized epilepsy treatment centers (e.g., Holmes et al., 1980) are likely to evaluate more patients who have both pseudoseizures and epileptic seizures, whereas general medical and psychological facilities are more likely to attract patients with acute or chronic conversion types of pseudoseizures. If one looks at the relationship from the opposite point of view, simultaneous EEG and video recording shows that the frequency of pseudoseizures among samples of epileptic patients is higher than was previously believed (Desai, Porter, & Penry, 1982). Williams et al. (1978) noted that medications do a good job of controlling 60% of all seizures. The remaining 40% include, in unknown proportions, intractable epileptic seizures, seizures responsive to psychological factors, and pseudoseizures. In the report by Holmes et al. (1980) of 53 children and adolescents with poorly controlled seizures, 3 (6%) definitely had pseudoseizures, 8 (15%) had both pseudoseizures and epileptic seizures, and another 8 (15%) were suspected of having pseudoseizures.

Many researchers have tried to link conversion symptoms with organic deficits (e.g., Whitlock, 1965) or cognitive deficits (e.g., Bendefeldt, Miller, & Ludwig, 1976). However, little work has been done on this connection as it applies specifically to pseudoseizures or to children. Sackellares et al. (1985) compared the cognitive performance of adult pseudoseizure patients with that of a group who had both epileptic seizures and pseudoseizures and with that of a group having epileptic seizures only. Although all groups showed some impairment, the cognitive functioning of the pseudoseizure group was less impaired than that of the other groups. The same underlying neurologic impairment is likely to cause both epileptic seizures and cognitive impairment. Thus, the epileptic's central nervous system substrate may be intrinsically more damaged as compared with that of the pseudoseizure group, who may also show neurologic deficit, but of a more subtle and insidious type. However, there is a problem in assessing cognitive deficits in any group of seizure patients. Anticonvulsant medications have detrimental effects on cognitive performance (Trimble, 1982), which may confound the results of some studies. For example, the epileptic seizure groups in the study of

Sackellares et al. (1985) had an earlier onset of symptoms and, thus, may have been receiving anticonvulsants for a longer period, which might partially account for their greater cognitive impairment.

Researchers still debate whether conversion symptoms are linked to as yet unidentified organic deficits. For example, Roy (1977) argued that in cases where such a link is found, it can be accounted for by the link between epilepsy and pseudoseizures, rather than by a more general organic factor in conversion symptoms. Whether the focus is on conversion symptoms or only on pseudoseizures, the existence of a link can be explained in either of two ways. The psychological explanation is in terms of secondary gain, whereby the patient with an organic deficit learns to play the "sick" role and then exaggerates or is unable to relinquish this role. The organic explanation is that an organic deficits exists, which produces both the symptoms of organicity and the symptoms of conversion. Trimble (1982) discussed evidence for a pattern of "antagonism" between pseudoseizures and epileptic seizures, which can be explained in terms of either secondary gain or a generalized organic deficit. Some individuals whose epileptic seizures are brought under control will subsequently develop pseudoseizures. We have described several children who fit this pattern, as has Williams et al. (1978).

Sexual Trauma

Although clinical experience and case reports suggest that sexual traumatization is associated with many cases of pseudoseizures, particularly among adolescent females, the statistical association of the two phenomena has not been well documented. In 1974, it was estimated that 90% of incest cases went unreported (Yates, 1982). This figure has probably changed somewhat, with new laws requiring helping professionals to report sexual abuse. However, the reluctance of many young women to admit that they have been molested still contributes to the difficulty in deriving accurate prevalence statistics.

The relationship between pseudoseizures and sexual trauma can be assessed either by studying the frequency of sexual trauma among pseudoseizure patients or the frequency of pseudoseizures among cases of sexual trauma. With regard to the former, Goodwin et al. (1979) found 4 cases of incest in a review of 12 cases of pseudoseizures. In compiling the histories of 21 pseudoseizure patients, without specifically soliciting information about sexual history, two cases of incest were revealed (Standage, 1975). Looking at the association in the alternative way, Davies (1978/1979) found six definite and two suspected cases of seizure disorder among 22 incest victims. However, Davies made no attempt to determine whether any of these were pseudoseizure cases. On the other hand, Browning and Boatman (1977) noted only one seizure disorder in 14 child incest victims that included 8 adolescent females. The degree of association will be hard to ascertain until larger samples of acute adolescent pseudoseizure cases and of incest victims have been studied and we have accurate estimates of the prevalence of incest in the general population.

How can this presumed association be explained? In their reports of small numbers of cases of adolescent females with pseudoseizures and histories of sexual trauma, several researchers have tried to uncover possible etiologic links. Gross (1979), who reported on four cases involving rape by the father or a father-surrogate, emphasized the continuing high level of anxiety that these young women experienced. This anxiety was related to both their fear that rape could recur and that it would be disclosed (on average, they kept the rape secret for a year), as well as feelings of guilt toward their mothers. Three of these four patients made suicidal gestures, suggesting how desperately they needed to escape from these pressures. LaBarbera and Dozier (1980) described evidence for a precise and continuing relationship between sexual trauma and pseudoseizures. In each of the four cases they reported, the initial pseudoseizure occurred in response to sexual molestation or some other traumatic sexual event. Subsequent pseudoseizures appeared in response to events that were in some way related to the initial event. For instance, one patient fainted while watching a health class film about sexual functioning, and another had a pseudoseizure during a therapy session while discussing her father's sexual abuse of her. This patient had a second pseudoseizure and had another one during a visit from her father. In each of their cases, LaBarbara and Dozier (1980) also presented evidence of a conflict regarding sexual matters, and pointed out that in at least one case, the initial "traumatic" event was not beyond the bounds of normal adolescent sexuality (such as initiating sexual behavior with a boyfriend), an observation Freud made almost 100 years ago (see Chapter 2).

Bernstein's (1969) report of three cases of pseudoseizures involving sexual "pressures" contains one case of sexual and physical abuse by the father, one case of an abnormally close father-daughter relationship but with no incest reported, and one case in which sexual conflicts existed but seemed unrelated to the father. In each case, pseudoseizures apparently stopped when the pressures were removed. The different types of sexual conflict that precipitated pseudoseizures in these three young women may reflect changes in clinicians' perseverance in uncovering incest and sexual abuse or it may indicate that sexual trauma and conflict need not always be a result of overt sexual abuse. Just as Freud pondered the relationship between and relative importance of real trauma, unresolved childhood fantasies, overstimulation in childhood, and constitutional deficits in hysteria, we and other researchers continue to consider them today.

Goodwin et al. (1979) described not only the guilt and anxiety of their patients, but also how pseudoseizures represent an ideal "choice" of symptom to express these feelings. Some victims of sexual abuse experience sexual excitement as well as rage, confusion, and shame; the pseudoseizure, often involving coital movements as well as the movements of resisting an attack, expresses both the exciting and the negative elements of their experience. Victims of sexual abuse also fear being controlled; the pseudoseizure reverses the situation because it frightens others and draws attention. In addition, the pseudoseizure can be the patient's way of revealing the abusive incident. If someone decodes the message implicit in their actions, they will be understood, but they are afraid to disclose it directly.

In each of these accounts, the pseudoseizure's function in releasing tension or anxiety is emphasized through disclosure, through dramatizing their predicament, or through repeating the traumatic experience. Pseudoseizures generally stop when the factors creating the anxiety have been alleviated. This suggests primary and secondary gain as the major explanation for the symptoms.

An interesting alternative view is suggested by Davies (1978/1979), who found a strong association between abnormal EEGs and incest. Seventeen (77%) of 22 incest victims had abnormal EEGs, compared with an overall incidence of 20% abnormal EEGs in that facility. Davies discussed the possibility that organic deficits related to these abnormal EEGs may also make these children more prone to becoming involved in deviant sexual relationships. This argument can be taken one step further; a general or specific organic-emotional vulnerability may exist, which predisposes individuals to both incest and pseudoseizures or other forms of psychopathology.

Treatment

Pseudoseizures can be treated using approaches similar to those used for other conversion symptoms. This section will summarize the essential components of treatment and management reported to be effective with pseudoseizures in childhood and adolescence, and will point out some special considerations for each subtype of pseudoseizure.

Clinicians who treat and manage pseudoseizures agree on several points. First, psychological factors should be brought under consideration earlier in the course of the evaluation and treatment rather than later. The physician who first sees the patient is better able to plan an evaluation if he or she is well informed about the differences between pseudoseizures and epileptic seizures and about the usual features of a conversion disorder. Psychological factors can be assessed concomitantly with organic factors. Friedman (1973) stressed that psychological investigation should not be used as a last resort; the physician's distrust of psychological influences only reinforces the patient's and family's distrust of psychological explanations. As a way of allaying this fear and distrust, Oberfield, Reuben and Burkes (1983) recommend an interdisciplinary approach, involving nonpsychiatric and psychiatric team members from the beginning.

A second point on which most clinician's agree is that the diagnosis of conversion disorder must be clearly stated and explained to the patient and family. This helps to avoid misinterpretations about the disorder's psychological nature. The difference between malingering and conversion should be explained so that the patient and family understand that the patient is not in conscious control of the seizures (Oberfield et al., 1983). In the case of pseudoseizures, and particularly in cases involving both pseudoseizures and epileptic seizures, the patient and family need to understand the difference between the two types of seizures. Ramani and Gumnit (1982) recommend a simple explanation about the relationship between pseudoseizures and stress. Getting a clear statement of the diagnosis on record also prevents further medical procedures, always a danger in conversion disorder. Since anticonvulsants will need to be reduced or withdrawn in pseudoseizure cases, the patient and family need a clear explanation of why these pills, to which they may have ascribed great powers, are no longer necessary.

Williams et al. (1978) and Ramani and Gumnit (1982) noted that a gamut of psychological interventions have been successful in treating pseudoseizures. Treatment needs to be planned on an individual basis so that the technique or combination of techniques most likely to benefit each individual is used. The following four components are essential to all treatments: (a) the patient is encouraged to talk about stress and conflicts as an alternative to using symptoms to communicate (Friedman, 1973); (b) the patient is taught simple coping strategies (Ramani & Gumnit, 1982); (c) where possible the pressures precipitating the pseudoseizures are removed; and (d) the contingencies of reinforcement that maintain and encourage the occurrence of seizures are changed.

1. *Encouraging the patient to talk about conflicts*. With younger children, play or projective techniques are appropriate. With older children and adolescents supportive/educative therapy or short-term dynamic psychotherapy works well. Family counseling may also facilitate communication about stress. A sexual abuse victim will often be encouraged to break his or her secrecy. Caldwell and Stewart (1981) used hypnosis to help an adolescent boy with pseudoseizures divulge information about being raped.

2. *Teaching simple coping strategies*. Communicating openly may also be considered a coping strategy. Other behavioral and cognitive strategies should be tailored to the patient's age, personality, and intelligence. With younger children, suggesting alternate behaviors may be most appropriate, whereas adolescents can be helped to achieve a perspective on their feelings and to be more assertive. In sexual abuse cases, this may be particularly relevant. Various forms of therapy are indicated here, including psychodynamic psychotherapy and relaxation and self-hypnosis techniques.

3. *Removal of pressures where possible*. When sexual abuse is a factor, legal authorities must be notified and the child or adolescent may have to be removed from a noxious home situation. More often, family members and the patient need to be counseled regarding appropriate behavior and how to respond effectively to inappropriate behavior. School and achievement pressures and problems with peers are other pressures that often need to be addressed through either therapy or a casework approach.

4. *Changing the contingencies of reinforcement*. The family must often be instructed about secondary gain, and taught to avoid giving the patient special attention when seizures occur. Suggesting ways of rewarding other behaviors

may also be helpful. With younger children or with patients whose IQs are low, an operant conditioning program may be useful in encouraging more positive forms of behavior. Adolescents and older children may be helped more when the benefits of being seizure-free are pointed out (for instance, being included in more activities or being able to learn to drive). However, if the adolescent needs the symptom for pressing emotional reasons, logical explanations may have limited efficacy.

The emphasis in treating each of the three subtypes of pseudoseizures is likely to be different. Children who have both pseudoseizures and epileptic seizures need to be told in simple terms that some of their seizures are related to stress, whereas others are not, and that they can act to control the stress-related seizures. Family members can be taught to recognize the differences between the two types of seizures and respond to each differently.

When the acute conversion type of pseudoseizure is treated in cases where sexual trauma or conflict is suspected, the patient is encouraged to disclose information about the traumatic episode and talk about the feelings it caused. Steps must be taken to prevent further sexual abuse. The patient is instructed in appropriate ways to set limits, seek help, and understand and cope with sexual feelings. An important component of the treatment of the sexually abused child is to help them ventilate all their feelings. The child often feels reluctant to discuss anger or ambivalent feelings. In addition, when there were some positive feelings about the perpetrator or some aspect of their relationship, the child may be particularly hesitant to express these sentiments. If a therapist considers some feelings unacceptable, the child may comply and not express those feelings. The therapist must be willing to hear all the child's feelings, accept them all as valid, and help the child come to terms with the confusing and conflicting feelings that sexual abuse arouses.

When pseudoseizures are part of a chronic polysymptomatic clinical picture, short-term treatment or crisis intervention is likely to fail. The clinician must make special efforts to develop an alliance with the patient and family, who are likely to be extremely resistant to psychological interpretations of seizures and other symptoms. The patient and family are likely to reject psychotherapeutic intervention if offered; when it is suggested, they may seek organic medical treatment elsewhere. For that reason, such cases are best treated in a medical context. The concept of stress-related symptoms should be introduced in a gradual nonthreatening way. Because these families often have an entrenched "somatic style" of communication and need the patient to remain in the sick role, treating only the patient's symptom often fails. While more intensive family therapy is often recommended, the family usually refuses it.

Although various modalities are recommended to treat chronic polysymptomatic disorders with pseudoseizures, no one has yet demonstrated empirically that any particular treatment is superior. Each clinician must decide what intervention is appropriate in each individual case, taking the patient's and the family's motivation into account.

Conclusions

Several points must be kept in mind to diagnose and effectively treat pseudoseizures in children and adolescents. Pseudoseizures are frequently superimposed on organic disorders, especially epilepsy. No single criterion reliably distinguishes pseudoseizures from epileptic seizures; the entire clinical picture must be studied with attention to specific patterns of symptoms and signs. Electroencephalograms are particularly susceptible to misreading if precise patterns, possible alternative explanations, and the larger clinical picture are not given adequate consideration. One way to avoid unneeded diagnostic procedures and prevent protracted pediatric neurologic evaluations is to consider psychological factors from the outset and look for indications of a somatoform disorder. As Williams et al. (1978) pointed out, pseudoseizures can be effectively managed in some cases without a definitive differentiation between psychological and neurologic factors. In addition to individual psychotherapy, supportive/educative psychotherapy for the patient and family, self-control techniques, behavior modification, and a casework approach all can be useful in reducing or eliminating conditions that create and maintain the pseudoseizures. Different prognoses and treatment approaches are apppropriate for different subtypes of pseudoseizures.

Our understanding of pseudoseizures in children and adolescents, like our understanding of somatoform symptoms in general, remains sketchy. The recently developed technique of simultaneous telemetered EEG and video recording has allowed more precise behavioral and neurologic descriptions of pseudoseizures. Yet, the subtypes of pseudoseizures are not accurately delineated and the degree of association between pseudoseizures and various other factors, including sexual trauma, epilepsy, other organic illness, and other forms of psychopathology in the individual and family, have yet to be established. How psychological factors are translated into neurologic or pseudoneurologic symptoms remains unknown. As a first step to developing hypotheses about the mechanisms underlying conversion, more research on the cognitive and neuropsychological aspects of pseudoseizures and other conversion symptoms is needed.

References

Bendefeldt, F., Miller, L., & Ludwig, A. (1976). Cognitive performance in conversion hysterics. *Archives of General Psychiatry, 33*, 1250–1252.

Bernstein, N.R. (1969). Psychogenic seizures in adolescent girls. *Behavioral Neuropsychiatry, 1*, 31–34.

Browning, D., & Boatman, B. (1977). Incest: Children at risk. *American Journal of Psychiatry, 134*, 69–73.

Caldwell, T., & Stewart, R. (1981). Hysterical seizures and hypnotherapy. *The American Journal of Clinical Hypnosis, 23*, 294–298.

Cohen, R., & Suter, C. (1982). Hysterical seizures: Suggestion as a provocative EEG test. *Annals of Neurology, 11*, 391–395.

Davies, R. (1978/1979). Incest: Some neuropsychiatric findings. *International Journal of Psychiatry in Medicine, 9*, 117–121.

Desai, B., Porter, R., & Penry, J. (1982). Psychogenic seizures: A study of 42 attacks in six patients with intensive monitoring. *Archives of Neurology, 39*, 202–209.

Dubowitz, V., & Hersov, L. (1976). Management of children with nonorganic (hysterical) disorders of motor function. *Developmental Medicine and Child Neurology, 18*, 358–368.

Finlayson, R., & Lucas, A. (1979). Pseudoepileptic seizures in children and adolescents. *Mayo Clinic Proceedings, 54*, 83–87.

Friedman, S. (1973). Conversion symptoms in adolescents. *Pediatric Clinics of North America, 20*, 873–882.

Goodwin, J., Simms, M., & Bergman, R. (1979). Hysterical seizures, sequel to incest. *American Journal of Orthopsychiatry, 49*, 698–703.

Goodyer, I. (1985). Epileptic and pseudoepileptic seizures in childhood and adolescence. *Journal of the American Academy of Child Psychiatry, 24*, 3–9.

Gross, M., (1979). Incestuous rape—a cause for hysterical seizures in four adolescent girls. *American Journal of Orthopsychiatry, 49*, 704–708.

Gross, M., & Huerta, E. (1980). Functional convulsions masked as epileptic disorders. *Journal of Pediatric Psychology, 3*, 71–79.

Guze, S., Woodruff, R., & Clayton, P. (1971). A study of conversion symptoms in psychiatric out-patients. *American Journal of Psychiatry, 128*, 645–646.

Holmes, G.L., Sackellares, J.C., McKiernan, J., Ragland, M., & Dreifuss, F.E. (1980). Evaluation of childhood pseudoseizures using EEG telemetry and videotape monitor. *Journal of Pediatrics, 97*, 554–558.

Konikow, N. (1983). Hysterical seizures or pseudoseizures. *Journal of Neurosurgical Nursing, 15*, 22–25.

Krumholtz, A., & Niedermeyer, E. (1983). Psychogenic seizures: A clinical study with follow-up data. *Neurology, 33*, 498–502.

LaBarbera, J., & Dozier, H. (1980). Hysterical seizures: The role of sexual exploitation. *Psychosomatics, 21*, 897–903.

Ljungberg, L. (1957). Hysteria: A clinical, prognostic, and genetic study. *Acta Psychiatrica Scandinavica*, (Suppl 112), 1–162.

Maloney, M.J. (1980). Diagnosing hysterical conversion reaction in childhood. *Journal of Pediatrics, 97*, 1016–1019.

Massey, E. (1982). History of epilepsy and hysteria. In T. Riley & A. Roy (Eds.). *Pseudoseizures* (pp. 1–18). Baltimore: Williams & Wilkins.

Masson, J.M. (1985). *The assault on truth: Freud's suppression of the seduction theory.* New York: Penguin.

Nicoll, J.S. (1981). Pseudoseizures: A neuropsychiatric diagnostic dilemma. *Psychosomatics, 22*, 451–454.

Niedermeyer, E., Blumer, D., Holscher, E., & Walker, B.A. (1970). Classical hysterical seizures facilitated by anticonvulsant toxicity. *Psychiatrica Clinica, 3*, 71–84.

Oberfield, R., Reuben, R., & Burkes, L. (1983). Interdisciplinary approach to conversion disorders in adolescent girls. *Psychosomatics, 24*, 983–989.

Ramani, V., & Gumnit, R. (1982). Management of hysterical seizures in epileptic patients. *Archives of Neurology, 39*, 78–81.

Rosenfeld, A.A (1979). Incidence of a history of incest among 18 female psychiatric patients. *American Journal of Psychiatry, 136*, 791–795.

Rosenfeld, A.A, Nadelson, C.C., & Krieger, M.J. (1979). Fantasy and reality in patients' reports of incest. *Journal of Clinical Psychiatry, 40*, 159–164.

Roy, A. (1977). Cerebral disease and hysteria. *Comprehensive Psychiatry, 18*, 607–609.

Roy, A. (1979). Hysterical seizures. *Archives of Neurology, 36*, 447.

Sackellares, J., Giordani, B., Seidenberg, M., Dreifuss, F.E., Vanderzant, C.W., & Boll, T.J. (1985). Patients with pseudoseizures: Intellectual and cognitive performance. *Neurology, 35*, 116–119.

Schneider, S., & Rice, D. (1979). Neurological manifestations of childhood hysteria. *Journal of Pediatrics, 94*, 153–156.

Scott, D. (1982). Recognition and diagnostic aspects of nonepileptic seizures. In T. Riley & A. Roy (Eds.), *Pseudoseizures* (pp. 21–33). Baltimore: Williams & Wilkins.

Silver, L. (1982). Conversion disorder with pseudoseizures in adolescence: A stress reaction to unrecognized and untreated learning disabilities. *Journal of the American Academy of Child Psychiatry, 21*, 508–512.

Standage, K.F. (1975). The etiology of hysterical seizures. *Canadian Journal of Psychiatry, 20*, 67–73.

Trimble, M. (1978). Serum prolactin in epilepsy and hysteria. *British Medical Journal, 13*, 1682.

Trimble, M. (1982). Anticonvulsant drugs and hysterical seizures. In T. Riley & A. Roy (Eds.), *Pseudoseizures* (pp. 148–158). Baltimore: Williams & Wilkins.

Whitlock, F.A. (1965). The aetiology of hysteria. *Acta Psychiatrica Scandinavica, 43*, 144–162.

Williams, D., & Mostofsky, D. (1982). Psychogenic seizures in childhood and adolescence. In T. Riley & A. Roy (Eds.), *Pseudoseizures* (pp. 169–184). Baltimore: Williams & Wilkins.

Williams, D., Spiegel, H., & Mostofsky, D. (1978). Neurogenic and hysterical seizures in children and adolescents: Differential diagnostic and therapeutic considerations. *American Journal of Psychiatry, 135*, 82–86.

Yates, A. (1982). Children eroticized by incest. *American Journal of Psychiatry, 139*, 482–485.

10

Conclusions

What do the available data tell us about the diagnosis of childhood somatoform disorders? Somatoform symptoms occur frequently in normal as well as disturbed children. Children with persistent symptoms and stable somatoform syndromes regularly see primary care practitioners, and are sometimes referred to pediatric neurologists or child psychologists and child psychiatrists. Despite the frequent occurrence of somatoform symptoms, full blown somatoform disorders occur so infrequently in children that a new diagnostic nomenclature was needed to replace DSM III criteria, which are too strict when applied to children. In addition, childhood somatoform disorders differ from those in adults. Childhood symptoms are more unstable; gender differences are less pronounced in early childhood, and children seem to have greater awareness of the psychological factors producing the symptom.

We have proposed a new nomenclature made up of descriptive syndromes that take into account the fluid nature and varying presentations of somatoform symptoms in childhood. This proposed nomenclature includes four categories of somatoform disorder.

Type 1 is a syndrome that describes children with many somatoform symptoms of a nonspecific but persistent type. These children come from families that give them secondary gain for their illnesses. However, the child's illness lacks a specific antecedent event, and no severe pervasive family psychopathology can be found. In the Type 1 disorder, the symptom is an adaptive strategy for coping with stress, but may progress to a more serious somatization disorder when the child experiences a serious stressor or if no intervention is forthcoming.

Type 2 is a syndrome that describes children with a single persistent physical symptom in which a stressor or precipitating event can be identified. The families of patients demonstrate a pathologic pattern of somatization that includes giving secondary gain for somatoform symptoms. In many such cases, the child's symptoms may help the entire family to avoid stress.

Type 1 (polysymptomatic) and Type 2 (monosymptomatic) disorders are new descriptive categories. They are working formulations that need further careful refinement and must be tried out in the field, using cross-validation studies to determine whether they are useful clinically. Many of these "not fully formed" somatization disorders may well be precursors of adult conversion reactions and somatization disorders. Further research is needed to test this hypothesis.

Children with the Type 3 syndrome often meet the criteria for DSM III conversion reaction. Both primary and secondary gain are present. A stressor often precedes the development of these symptoms. In some cases, the symptoms may have a specific symbolic meaning. Some of the children seem unconcerned about their symptom (*la belle indifférence*).

Type 4 is a polysymptomatic disorder that closely approximates adult somatization disorder. The patient has multiple persistent symptoms, often of a more general sort (not just pseudoneurologic), and sometimes with an accompanying personality disorder. However, these children often do not meet DSM III criteria because due to their age, they lack the requisite number of symptoms.

What do we know about the characteristics of children with somatoform symptoms? We know that children with such symptoms come from families with poor ability to express many types of feelings. The child who somatizes often has a model in their environment who uses somatoform symptoms as a coping strategy. We also know sexual stressors are frequent antecedents, particularly in some symptoms like pseudoseizures. In adolescent females, these symptoms and sexual stressors often occur concurrently; in some cases, sexual stress appears to be the primary etiologic factor.

The correlation of early sexual abuse with later psychopathology and specifically with conversion symptoms is far from perfect. We do not subscribe to the theory that conversion disorders always and inevitably result from sexual abuse. In our view, whether such antecedents are specific to somatoform disorders or associated with psychiatric disorder as a general rule still has not been clearly delineated. We have seen many abused children who have not developed somatoform disorders and other children with conversion symptoms who have suffered other psychological traumata. What role sexual overstimulation short of abuse plays in causing these conditions remains an intriguing research question.

The psychological and physiologic precursors of somatoform symptoms are not well understood. Although psychoanalytic explanations of conversion reactions are plentiful, far more empiric study is needed to support or refute them. Other theories about the etiology of somatoform disorders are not well articulated. Perhaps we are groping for ways to understand a puzzle that has intrigued behavioral scientists since Charcot, Meynart, and Freud. How are psyche and soma related? By what mechanism can psychological factors give rise to physical symptoms? What constitutes a predisposing factor and how do they contribute to the development of somatoform symptoms? Previously, "constitutional predisposition" was a concept used to explain what could not be attributed to environmental factors.

The relationship of specific predispositional states to the development of somatoform symptoms is beginning to be studied. Genetic factors are beginning to emerge, particularly in polysymptomatic disorders. Studies of sensory inhibition, alexithymia, disconnection syndromes, and other neuropsychological and neurophysiologic studies, although few, are gaining increasing attention in explaining adult disorders. Children with somatoform symptoms have been found to have a higher incidence of learning problems than do children with other psychiatric symptoms, perhaps indicating some sort of associated but undefined cognitive deficit. Empiric studies of associated personality characteristics, the use of various defensive strategies, and the function of somatoform symptoms are sorely needed. We need to know how somatoform symptoms emerge at various stages of the child's emotional, social, and cognitive development. What is their natural history? What variables alter their developmental course?

What do we know about treatment? Because cases of childhood somatoform disorders present more commonly to the primary care physician, being familiar with management strategies and referral procedures can avert more serious psychopathology by early diagnosis and proper family intervention. However, in many cases, the child should be referred to mental health practitioners.

Most experts recommend a two-step procedure to treat somatoform disorders. We feel that this approach is particularly appropriate in monosymptomatic disorders. Symptom removal using such techniques as hypnosis, direct suggestion, and biofeedback is the first step. Biofeedback seems particularly helpful in children with headache, where its efficacy without other accompanying interventions has been demonstrated. However, some children who need their symptoms for pressing psychological reasons may become quite anxious if the symptom is removed. Every case must be evaluated to determine whether a simultaneous decrease in stress may be critical in maintaining the symptom removal.

The second step in treatment is removing or ameliorating the stress causing or sustaining the symptom. This may be accomplished through environmental changes, individual psychotherapy, and parental counseling.

In difficult cases, especially in somatization disorders, psychological treatment is often ineffective because family psychopathology is too severe or entrenched. Careful management and symptomatic treatment are often all that can be done. In severe cases, the child sometimes must be removed from the home. Many discussions of such cases recommend family therapy as an alternative. This form of treatment is currently popular and would seem to be the logical choice. However, so little objective data and so few carefully done outcome studies are available that we doubt that the current enthusiasm is based on empiric review of treatment success. Our own experience is that such families are usually too resistant to treat with this modality.

Although follow-up studies of children with conversion reactions suggest that the acute symptoms resolve, long-term outcomes are uncertain. These children may continue to be at risk for future symptoms when they experience stress. We need to know if early intervention prevents possible debilitating deterioration in somatization disorder. Longitudinal studies are greatly needed.

Children with somatoform disorders rarely appear in the mental health setting. Many psychologists and psychiatrists know very little about these disorders. Thus, appropriate referrals, competent management, and effective treatment are sometimes hard to find. Both the clinician and the clinical researcher in psychiatry and psychology need to become integrated members of the pediatric team. In this way, children with somatoform disorders will be better understood and more effectively treated.

Author Index

Subject Index

MIX
Papier aus verantwortungsvollen Quellen
Paper from responsible sources
FSC® C105338

If you have any concerns about our products,
you can contact us on
ProductSafety@springernature.com

In case Publisher is established outside the EU,
the EU authorized representative is:
Springer Nature Customer Service Center GmbH
Europaplatz 3, 69115 Heidelberg, Germany

Printed by Libri Plureos GmbH
in Hamburg, Germany